How to Write a Grant Application

How to Write a Grant Application

Allan Hackshaw

Deputy Director
Cancer Research UK & UCL Cancer Trials Centre
University College London
London, UK

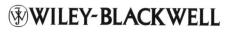

WILEY-BLACKWELL

A John Wiley & Sons, Ltd., Publication

BMJ|Books

Library of Congress Cataloging-in-Publication Data

Hackshaw, Allan K.
    How to write a grant application / Allan Hackshaw.
        p. ; cm.
    Includes bibliographical references and index.
    ISBN 978-1-4051-9755-7 (alk. paper)
  1. Proposal writing in medicine. 2. Medicine—Research grants. 3.
Proposal writing for grants. I. Title.
    [DNLM: 1. Research Support as Topic. 2. Biomedical Research. 3.
Writing—standards.   W 20.5]
    R853.P75H33 2011
    610.79—dc22

                                                                                          2010036482

A catalogue record for this book is available from the British Library.

This book is published in the following electronic formats: ePDF 9781444329667; Wiley Online Library 9781444329650; ePub 9781444329674

Set in 9.5/12pt Minion by MPS Limited, a Macmillan Company, Chennai, India

Printed and bound in Malaysia by Vivar Printing Sdn Bhd

1   2011

Contents

Foreword

Writing a grant is often a painstaking process. However, if one is fortunate it can be aided by an experienced mentor who has learnt over many years how to navigate through the complex process of taking a scientific hypothesis from an idea to a formal proposal that leads to a financially viable set of experiments or studies. For most aspiring academic clinicians or scientists, career development depends on publishing their scientific work. Obtaining grant funding even in a buoyant economy is never easy. As financial pressure on government, industries and charities increases, the chance of successful funding diminishes.

In *How to write a Grant Application* the author brings together many years experience of obtaining grants for clinical and scientific projects. Allan Hackshaw provides an invaluable resource to guide the reader through each step in the preparation, writing and management of a grant.

Regulations concerning the conduct of clinical trials in humans are complex and have created a new terminology that needs to be understood and incorporated into grant applications. The book describes the important components that need to be considered in formulating a grant application that will lead to a study that is scientifically sound, realistic and feasible.

Each section of the book will help the reader formulate a logical and clear application covering the scientific, financial and administrative components needed to run a modern series of experiments or a clinical study. By reading this book the applicant should be able to avoid the common pitfalls involved in writing a grant so that more time can be spent crafting a mature scientific application that is internationally competitive.

Professor Jonathan A Ledermann
Director, Cancer Research and UCL Cancer Trials Centre,
University College London

Preface

All researchers are familiar with how most projects, and the people who work on them, are funded. A large majority of projects need to be funded from specific study grants that must be applied for in a competitive fashion, including training fellowships and doctoral studentships. Many applications are not successful due to a variety of problems, some of which could have been avoided in the submitted application or by having a better understanding of the review process and what is usually expected by the funding committee and their external reviewers. Funding organisations want value for money, and because there are many researchers applying for a limited pool of funds, applicants need to develop and write a strong and well-written application, so that it is likely to be ranked above most of the others, and therefore successfully funded.

This book aims to provide a clear account of how to develop a grant application that hopefully will have a better chance of success. It will cover the key aspects of writing a grant application, namely describing the justification, feasibility and value of the proposed study; the design, and being clear about objectives, hypotheses and outcomes; estimating financial costs; and a description of a typical funding committee review process. The book also distinguishes between the different types of studies (observational studies, clinical trials and laboratory experiments).

Allan Hackshaw
Deputy Director,
Cancer Research UK & UCL Cancer Trials Centre

Acknowledgements

I would like to express many thanks to those who commented on draft chapters: Kerry Chester, Cheryl Mason Rosalind Raine and Jane Wooders. I am most grateful to Jan Mackie for her careful and thorough editing. Final thanks go to Harald Bauer.

About the author

Allan Hackshaw has been working in academic clinical research since 1991, with experience in a variety of areas including smoking and health, antenatal and cancer screening, and treatments for several disorders including cancer and migraine. He has been co-investigator on many successful grant applications to public sector bodies, charities or commercial organisations; with a total funding amount of over £24.7 million associated with observational studies, clinical trials and systematic reviews. Just as importantly, he has also been involved in unsuccessful applications and learnt key lessons from the experience. He has acted as an external reviewer for grant funding bodies, and been a member of one of the main funding committees at Cancer Research UK (Clinical Trials Advisory Awards Committee, CTAAC) since 2007.

Chapter 1 **Overview**

Many researchers in health sciences need to obtain funding in order to establish or continue with their work. This is a common activity in the non-commercial (academic or public) sector, such as universities and hospital research departments. The process of obtaining financial support is usually very competitive, particularly when there are limited resources. Funding bodies also need to ensure that their grants will be put to the best use, maximising the effect on clinical practice, public health, scientific knowledge or future research.

It can easily take 1–2 years (often more) from inception of a research proposal until the first subject is recruited to the study. This may sometimes feel daunting to researchers, especially those new to the field. However, as more people become involved and time is spent on developing the idea and study design, the likelihood of it being successfully funded should increase. If it has been thought through properly, major potential problems and design issues will have been considered and addressed in the application, rather than being raised for the first time by the funding committee or its external reviewers. It can be easy for experienced reviewers to distinguish a polished and cogent application that may have taken perhaps several months to develop and write, from one that has been written hastily in 3 weeks and only seen by one or two colleagues.

There is no such thing as a perfect grant application. The external reviewers and funding committee will usually have criticisms, and the applicants themselves often see ways of improving their application with hindsight. What largely matters is making the proposed project look important enough to be funded, that it is well designed, and that the financial costs are reasonable.

How to Write a Grant Application, 1st edition. © Allan Hackshaw. Published 2011 by Blackwell Publishing Ltd.

1.1 Types of grants

Grants are used to investigate a multitude of study objectives:
- Examining risk factors for or causes of disease or early death.
- Examining the characteristics, attitudes, experiences or behaviour of defined groups of people.
- Evaluating methods for preventing, detecting or treating disease, or preventing early death.
- Laboratory experiments on biological samples, animals or simple organisms, in order to investigate the effects of a stimulus or exposure, identify associations, or as part of drug development.
- Correlating biological measurements with each other, or with patient outcomes, such as examining genetic, protein or other biomarkers associated with a disorder or early death.

The types of grants available to researchers include the following.

1.1.1 Project grants

These are the most common and are the type of grants with which researchers are familiar. The idea for a specific project is first thought of by one or two people in the field, who then establish a small group of colleagues to develop the idea further before applying for a grant. Alternatively, a project title can be first developed by a funding organisation, perhaps through an advisory committee, which has identified a need for a particular piece of research. The organisation advertises this (sometimes referred to as a *call for proposals*), and interested applicants then compete over who can address the research idea with the best study design and most acceptable resource requirements.

Project grants can cover any length of time, depending on the objectives, how common the disorder is and the number of expected participating centres. For example, a systematic review of a set of 10 published clinical trials, that involves obtaining raw data from each trial group, could take 12–18 months to complete, whereas a screening trial to identify people at a high risk of stomach cancer and to prevent it through adequate treatment could take over 10 years. An early phase clinical treatment trial of 50 patients could run for 2 years, compared with a late phase randomised trial of 500 patients that could take around 5 years.

1.1.2 Fellowships and doctoral (research) postgraduate degrees

These usually fund either a specific person who has formulated a research idea as part of his/her professional development, or a project proposal that has been advertised by a research department. Fellowships, which are competitive, are a sign of personal professional achievement if the grant application is successful.

They can be awarded to those who are already employed and the grant will allow the recipient to focus their research on a particular area for a fixed time period. Doctoral research degrees are common, particularly among people who are early in their career. The study objectives for these two types of grants are similar to those for project grants but are often smaller-scale studies, limited to laboratory experiments, or involving only a few centres for studies of humans, because funding is for a fixed length of time, for example 3–5 years.

1.1.3 Programme grants

Programme grants apply to a set of related projects in a particular field of research. These could fund a group of people with a common general research goal, or may support the formation of a core unit, either on its own or as part of a larger department, for example, establishing a clinical trials unit to design and conduct treatment trials in particular disorder. A programme grant can also be used to fund a set of new related studies to examine aspects of a disorder, for example, looking at different risk factors for heart disease, such as lifestyle characteristics, genetic and biological markers in blood or urine. These types of grants involve significant amounts of money and are associated with a duration of several years, for example 5 or 10 years, sometimes with the expectation that the grant will be renewed at the end of the period. Those who lead the units supported by these grants usually have prior experience with securing project grants and are established in their field of research.

Each of these three types of grants requires different levels of effort spent in the application process; the input is approximately in proportion to the funding requested. Programme grants are the most intensive to prepare because they are expensive, they will employ several people and last for many years. Project grants are perhaps the most competitive because they are usually open to any level of researcher, ie. those new to the field or already established. Grants for fellowships and research degrees tend to be offered by relatively few organisations, such as governmental research councils or charitable bodies, and are for short periods of time (up to about 3–5 years). These grants may be relatively easier to obtain, but elements of the grant application are similar to project grants.

1.2 Types of funding organisations

Several types of organisations provide funding for research projects:
- *Governmental bodies or research councils*
  - Department of Health/National Health Service (UK)
  - Medical Research Council (UK)
  - National Institutes of Health (USA) (see Yang 2005 for specific details about applying for NIH grants)

- National Cancer Institute (USA)
- Biotechnology and Biological Sciences Research Council (UK)
- *Regional or international funding organisations*
  - European Research Council
  - European Commission
  - Association for International Cancer Research
  - World Health Organization
- *Charities, disease-specific associations or foundations*
  - British Heart Foundation (UK)
  - Cancer Research UK (UK)
  - March of Dimes (USA)
  - Bill and Melinda Gates Foundation
  - Deutsche Forschungsgemeinschaft (DFG, German Research Foundation)
- *Local trustees within an organisation*: Some hospitals have a trustees' fund, which has accumulated from donations made by former or current employees, or by patients. Such funds are usually available to conduct relatively small-scale studies within that organisation (i.e. local or single centre studies), and not usually with national or international centres.
- *Commercial companies*: Some pharmaceutical companies and those that manufacture medical devices often provide funds to researchers in the non-commercial sector (e.g. a university), to conduct a clinical trial using one of their products. The drug or medical device may or may not already be licensed for use in humans, but it is almost always provided to the researchers without any cost. In some instances, the company also gives financial support to set up and conduct the trial in the form of a study-specific grant or an educational grant.
- *Private benefactors*: A researcher or research unit may have developed a professional relationship with a single, relatively wealthy individual who is willing to support them for a specific project. It is often the case that the benefactor (or his/her family member) has suffered from an illness related to the work of the researcher.

There is also a website called researchresearch.com that lists a wide range of funding organisations, including many of the smaller ones. The website is http://new.researchresearch.com.

Almost all grant applications will be considered by a funding committee, a group of experts with various backgrounds who are internal or external to the funding organisation. They will make the decision to fund a study or not.

Each funding organisation has its own process for grant applications. It is not the purpose of this book to cover specific agencies, nor to compare and contrast between them. However, the information required from prospective researchers and many elements of the review process tend to be very similar, particularly for the larger well-known funding bodies. Details of the application process for a particular organisation should be available from their website, the application form or other documentation sent on request. Many regularly update their terms and conditions and requirements, so it is important to check these for each application as they may have changed since the last time the researcher submitted to the funding body. The organisation will usually have administrative staff available to provide advice on the application process by email or telephone.

Many application forms can be downloaded from the funding body's website (often in Microsoft Word), to be completed electronically and emailed or posted with the relevant signatures. Sometimes, there is an online submission form which is transferred directly to the funding body without the need for a hard copy (this is becoming increasingly common), though original signatures may still be expected to be posted.

1.3 Choosing an appropriate funding body

It will often be obvious which organisations are appropriate for funding a specific project, and large organisations sometimes have separate funding streams for different types of studies (such as laboratory experiments, observational studies or clinical trials). Colleagues with prior experience may recommend an appropriate funding body, or applicants could obtain information from websites or other documentation. When there are several potential funding organisations, the researcher needs to decide which might be the most appropriate after discussion with the Study Team (the group of people responsible for developing the study and who will usually be co-applicants; see Chapter 2). An application on the same topic should not be sent to more than one funding body at the same time with the expectation that this increases the chance of success. This is not usually allowed, and it avoids an unsatisfactory situation where two funding organisations approve the same study and applicants have to reject one.

Deciding which funding organisation to apply to may depend on the following factors:

- Whether there is a limit to the amount that can be requested, either each year or in total, or for single items of equipment.
- How wealthy the funding body is (small organisations are highly unlikely to fund large expensive studies).
- Whether or not the funding body will include institutional overheads (indirect costs) as part of the grant (see Section 6.2, page 82).
- Whether the application success rate for a funding body is low (usually because there are so many applications).

If the application is unsuccessful, it is always possible to submit a revised version elsewhere. However, the reviewers' comments should always be taken into account unless they are entirely inappropriate, because the next funding body may use one or more of the same reviewers. This may often be by chance, but is far more likely if the field of research is relatively narrow with a limited pool of appropriate experts.

1.4 Contents of the grant application

What is required from the applicants will usually be clear, either from the section headings in the application form itself or the guidelines from the funding organisation. Figure 1.1 provides an overview of the key features that are expected to be addressed in a typical grant application. Background, biological plausibility and justification, feasibility, and how the study results and conclusions will be used are covered in more detail in Chapter 3, while study design (which often forms most of the application) is discussed in Chapter 4. When there is no guidance from the funding body on the structure of the application (e.g. a commercial company or private benefactor), the main headings from Figure 1.1 could be used.

All projects should have a simple and concise title (one sentence). It is also worth creating an acronym for the study using letters from the title (sometimes the first letter from key words), or some word that encompasses the study aim, but check whether the same acronym is already in use for similar studies.

1.5 Including several studies in one application (project grants)

Most applications are associated with a single project, but there are occasions when several related projects are specified, though it is not meant to be a programme grant (see page 3). Sometimes, this approach is an efficient way to examine two or more objectives without having completely separate studies. For example, evaluating several treatments for a rare disorder as patients proceed through the clinical pathway from initial diagnosis to improvement, stable disease or progression, where different subsequent treatments are used according to level of recovery. Alternatively, there could be several related laboratory experiments, with specific but distinct stages.

Having too many sub-studies and objectives can make the application difficult to follow, or the overall project too complex. Occasionally, the funding committee may like parts of the project, but not others, and therefore need to decide whether to fund only these parts or decline the entire

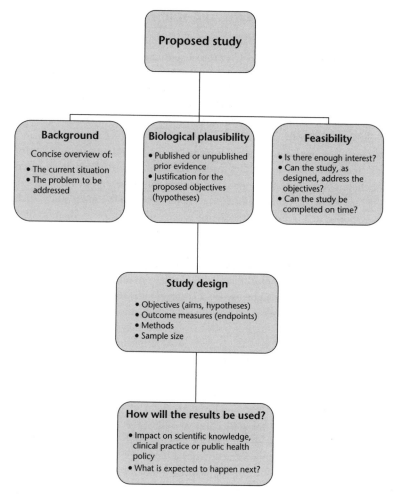

Figure 1.1 Key features of a typical grant application.

study. Applicants should, therefore, generally aim to avoid having too many sub-studies within a single application. If this approach is judged to be appropriate, applicants must provide a clear scientific justification, and show that there really is a central theme between the constituent studies. They will need to demonstrate that these are not different studies simply cobbled together. The applicants also need to ensure that one sub-study does not have an adverse impact on another, and that the results of any sub-study can be interpreted easily. A (simple) diagram showing how they all fit together would be helpful (see pages 38–39).

1.6 Translational research sub-studies

Many studies on humans, particularly case–control and cohort studies and clinical trials, will have clear objectives regarding a specific disorder or prevention of early death. However, it is becoming more common to collect biological samples as part of the main study, to be stored centrally in a laboratory for future, sometimes unspecified, analyses (i.e. the creation and maintenance of a *biobank*). This secondary analysis is sometimes referred to as a *translational research study*. The samples are usually blood, saliva or urine, but may also include tissue samples (e.g. cancerous tissue removed from affected patients). The analyses involve measuring biomarkers which could be chemical, biological (eg. genomic or proteomic markers) or radiological, that are to be correlated with clinical outcomes from the main study, such as response to a treatment, disease incidence, disease severity or mortality. Examples of this could be to examine the prognostic value of a biomarker (i.e. how well it correlates with a clinical outcome), its predictive value (i.e. whether the marker can be used to identify subgroups of individuals that are, for example, more likely to benefit from a certain treatment), or whether a biomarker can be used as a surrogate measure.

Adding a translational research sub-study could strengthen an application for the main study; the funding body may feel that they are getting more value for their money. Applicants may not need to describe in detail what the actual laboratory analyses will entail, because funding for the particular sub-study is sometimes applied for at a later date, or even from a different funding organisation. The application could briefly indicate the type of samples to be collected, when this will be undertaken, and whether there are any markers of current interest that would be measured. However, not all studies would benefit from having a translational study component, and indeed the collection and storage of biological samples could sometimes be a hindrance to the main study. The Study Team should decide together whether such a sub-study might be useful.

1.7 The application process

Figure 1.2 shows an overview of a typical grant application process (the funding committee evaluation is described in Chapter 7). Some funding bodies have an initial screening process for project grants, where an *outline application* is requested first and if there is sufficient interest, a subsequent *full application* is invited for the next committee meeting. Researchers should not underestimate the importance of an outline application. Although it is shorter and does not normally include details about the financial costs and collaborators, in reality the time and effort spent producing a well-written document may not be significantly less than that for a full application.

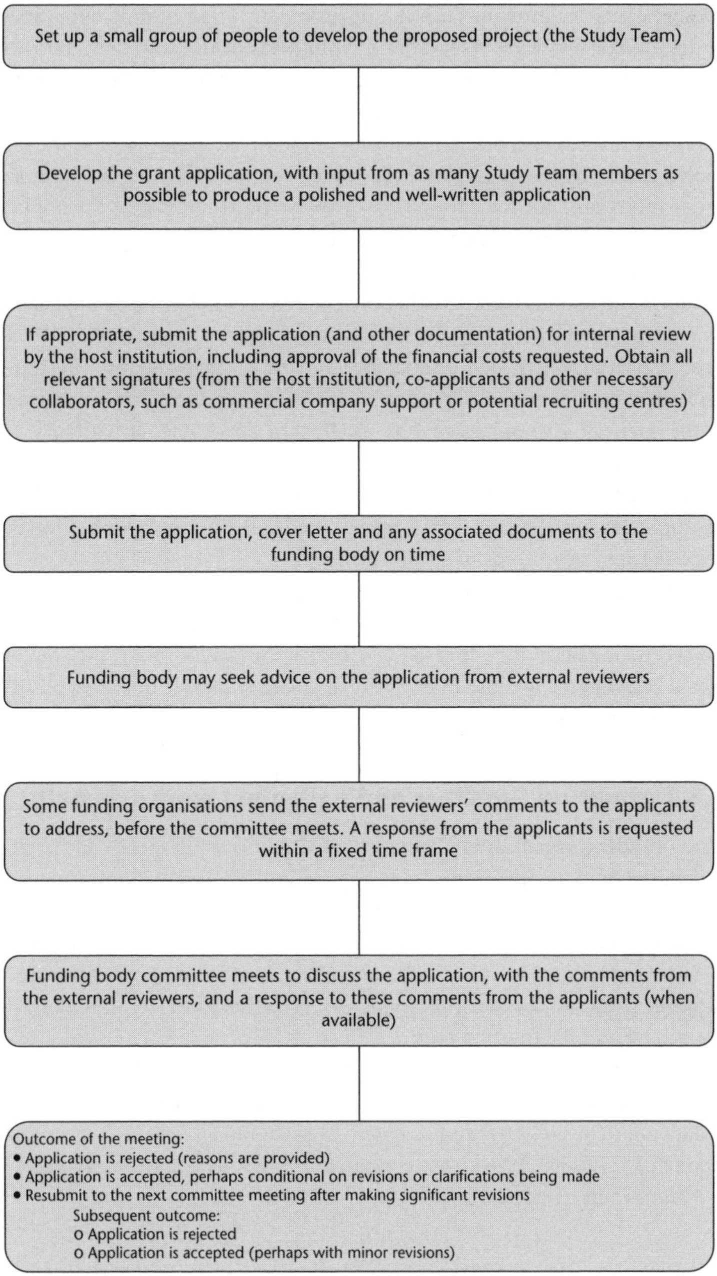

Figure 1.2 Overview of a typical grant application process.

Applicants occasionally rush the development of an outline application, and although they have reservations about parts of the text, they choose to submit anyway. There is little to be gained by this. It is likely that the review committee will have significant concerns and at best will request major revisions or clarifications, deferring consideration of the application to the next meeting. The applicants could have waited for the following meeting and spent more time on the application. A worse outcome is that the application is rejected outright, and there is no chance to revise the application and obtain funding.

Researchers should be aware that even before they submit their application to a funding body, it is often necessary for there to be an internal review by the host institution which will conduct the study, or act as the Sponsor in studies on humans (see Section 2.3, page 20). This review tends to focus on approval of the financial costs requested. It is usually signed by someone with financial authority, and the Head of Department.

Several other signatures may also be required, including those of all the co-applicants (see Section 2.1.1, page 19) and collaborators (see Section 5.4, page 76), and time needs to be allowed for this.

Almost all funding bodies have deadlines by which applications must be received.[1] Applicants should always submit their application on time. If there is likely to be a delay, the administrative staff at the funding body must be contacted beforehand, because in exceptional circumstances it might be possible to get an extension.

1.8 Estimating timelines and a planned work schedule

Many funding organisations request that the applicants specify the project *milestones* or *timescale* in the grant application. These are dates or periods during the course of the entire study over which certain tasks are expected to have been completed. Such schedules can only ever be approximate because unforeseen events, which often occur, can delay a project by several months. Estimated project milestones can nonetheless be useful to both the applicants and the funding body:

• They allow the applicants to see when certain tasks need to be completed, when different types of staff will be required and for how long, and when data are to be collected and analysed. This should all help with estimating the financial costs. It also gives applicants a rough schedule to work towards if successfully funded.

---

[1] Exceptions could be commercial companies who review project proposals frequently, for example every month.

- It allows the funding body to envisage a likely time frame for each part of the project, and to decide whether each section has an appropriate duration. If the grant is awarded, it is common for the funding body to request annual reports or updates from the researchers in order to determine whether the project is running on time, and if there are any major problems (see Section 8.1, page 115). These can be compared with the original milestones.

Box 1.1 shows typical parts of a project schedule. It does not have to be overly detailed, and need only indicate each major stage of the proposed study.

Box 1.1 Project milestones and possible associated activities		
Milestone	Main activity (will depend on the type of study)	Length of time (examples of what could be specified)
Study set-up	• Develop and finalise the study protocol, and any other relevant documents such as the Participant Information Sheet and consent forms (human studies). • Develop, submit and obtain all study approvals (national, local/institutional, ethics, regulatory, etc.). • Set up recruiting sites. • Order laboratory equipment or other materials. • Obtain animals, and prepare and implement procedures for housing and maintaining them.	Year 1 (6 months)

Study conduct	• Clinical trial in humans
	   • Identify and recruit subjects.
	   • Intervention period.
	   • Follow-up period.
	 • Observational studies of humans
	   • Identify and recruit subjects.
	   • Collect data (from questionnaires, interviews, hospital records, national databases, etc.).
	   • Follow-up period (cohort study).
		Years 1–4 (42 months); this could be divided further according to major activities. For example, in a clinical trial: Recruit subjects: 24 months Intervention: 6 months Follow-up: 12 months

(Continued)

Box 1.1 (Continued)		

Milestone	Main activity (will depend on the type of study)	Length of time (examples of what could be specified)

	• Laboratory experiments
	  • Develop the methodology.
	  • Prepare the experiments, instal equipment.
	  • Conduct the experiment.	

Data analysis	• First analysis – discuss with the Study Team. • Second analysis – revised or additional analyses, discuss again with the Study Team. • Final analysis.	Year 5 (12 months)
Report	• First draft – review by Study Team. • Final draft – after incorporating comments from the Study Team. • Final report submitted to funding body (when required).	Year 6 (3 months)
Dissemination	• Submit for presentation at conference and for submission to journal.	Year 6

1.9 Intellectual property

Occasionally a proposed laboratory experiment or clinical trial could lead to a product or method that can be patented. In this situation, the grant applicants will need to ascertain who owns the intellectual property. It could, for example, be split between the host institution, the funding body and the research unit. Details, such as how much each party receives from the patent earnings, should be discussed before an application is made, and may be finalised after an application is successfully awarded. There may be a specific section in the application form on intellectual property, and administrative staff at the funding body can usually help with this aspect. If the study is funded and sponsored by a commercial company, the company will usually own any intellectual property. If a commercial company provides funds to conduct the study but an academic institution is the Sponsor, an agreement would have to be made between these two organisations over the distribution of the patent, and this would be specified in a formal contract.

1.10 Text, grammar and format

It should be obvious that the text in a grant application should be easy to read, clear and where possible free from (or have limited) overly technical jargon. Also, abbreviations should be kept to a minimum, except those that are well-known and in common use in the field. Non-scientists will often be a member of the review committee for applications for studies on humans, and it is sometimes frustrating for them to try to understand exactly what the proposed study entails. Even technical laboratory experiments, which tend to be reviewed by like-minded experts, can benefit from simpler language in many sections of the application, where possible. Simplifying the text can indicate that the applicants know their subject matter well, because they can communicate to a high standard. This can improve the chance of success. Funding committees and external reviewers who struggle to understand an application will often cite this as a specific criticism. An application with many grammatical and spelling mistakes will appear unprofessional, and may be viewed negatively. The more people who have read and commented on the application prior to submission, the more likely that the application will read well.

The application form, or funding body guidelines, will specify the font size and other formatting characteristics, such as the preferred referencing system. The whole application should be examined before it is submitted to ensure, for example, that all the text has the same font size and that headings and numbered sections follow logically.

Applicants should aim to keep within the word or page limit for each section (if specified), but nevertheless avoid having an overly long application. The funding committee and external reviewers will have difficulty in reading through many pages of dense text. If the application is easy to read, the reviewers will understand and interpret the proposed project more readily, and this can indicate that the applicants have a good grasp of their study. It is best to have short paragraphs, avoid long sentences, and use subheadings in each section when appropriate, because this can greatly improve the structure of the application. For example, within a main section associated with the justification for a clinical trial of a new drug, subheadings for 'Biological mechanism', 'Prior evidence on efficacy' and 'Prior evidence on safety' could be created. Applicants should also identify if any repetitive statements are made within or between sections, and edit or remove them.

Some grant applications are improved by including tables or diagrams. These should be of good quality (i.e. high resolutions), and may often convey information in a clearer and more succinct way than using extensive text. Applicants need to ensure that the tables or diagrams are relevant to the proposal, are labelled properly, have clear legends and symbols, and if taken from published sources, are correctly referenced. Overly complex or detailed tables and diagrams are difficult to interpret and can hinder rather than aid the interpretation of the application. Colour illustrations might seem appealing, and in some cases are necessary, but applicants should bear in mind that the application will probably be printed in black and white. Some funding bodies send the application electronically to the committee and reviewers. Although this saves printing costs and items in colour can be seen on a computer screen, many reviewers still prefer to read through a hard copy and will therefore print them off anyway.

Summary points

- Know the application process and the timelines, including any prior internal approvals required by the host institution.
- Allow sufficient time to develop the application with several colleagues, so that the ideas can be considered carefully, major issues are identified and addressed, and the text looks well written.
- Do not have dense sections of text; use short paragraphs and short sentences, perhaps with section subheadings.
- Use simple tables and diagrams to summarise information or describe parts of the methods.
- Aim to have several versions of the application (at least five), with significant improvements between each revision.
- If the submission deadline is close, but the application has not been thoroughly evaluated or is not well written, consider waiting for the next deadline (if possible).
- If the text does not read well, or applicants themselves have concerns, do not submit and take a chance to see what happens, because this can look unprofessional and affect future applications; wait for the next deadline.
- Make sure that the current version of the application form from the funding organisation is used.
- Carefully read the instructions for submission from the funding body.
- Do not send the same application to more than one funding organisation at the same time.
- Do not combine several unrelated projects in the same application (unless specifically allowed).
- Contact administrative staff at the funding body over any general queries.
- Do not submit the application after the deadline has passed (even if by only a day), unless you have explicit permission to do so by the funding body.

Chapter 2 **People involved in the study**

Almost all projects require a team of people, and key members of the team together should design the study and write the application. These members are then directly involved in conducting the study, if it is successfully funded. In addition, there may be staff based at *centres* (or *sites*) in which study subjects are to be recruited, or experts who will provide a service or advice on a specific topic, but who do not have the same level of input as the grant applicants. For large studies, that are expected to have a significant impact on scientific knowledge, clinical practice or public health, there should be clear evidence of close collaboration between people from the different areas of expertise necessary for the study to succeed (see also Section 7.5.6, page 110).

2.1 Who should be part of the Study Team?

One of the most serious mistakes made by researchers applying for grants is that they do not develop the application with input from enough people, and that the draft has not been critically revised sufficiently to produce a polished application before submission. This often means that there are major problems with the study that are easily identified by the funding committee or its external reviewers, which should have been addressed by the grant applicants.

There are various terms used to label the group of people that has responsibility for a particular project, i.e. the design, conduct and interpretation of the results. These are:
- Study Team.
- Study or Trial Management Group.
- Study or Trial Steering Committee.[1]

---

[1] In some places 'Trial Steering Committee' is an independent committee that acts on behalf of the funding organisation and helps to oversee the trial.

How to Write a Grant Application, 1st edition. © Allan Hackshaw. Published 2011 by Blackwell Publishing Ltd.

The choice of label sometimes depends on geographical location. Most, if not all, of the key people on the study team should be *co-applicants* or *co-investigators*, in order to provide different areas of expertise, which are necessary to conduct the study successfully. They are named on the grant application, and therefore have some formal ownership of the study, and are expected to be authors of the associated publications. The lead applicant (investigator) is often called the *Chief Investigator*: the key researcher for the study and often the person who first developed the idea (Box 2.1). He/she will lead the Study Team. Almost all grant applications require a single named chief investigator, and it is not common to have co-chief investigators. Some funding bodies require the Chief Investigator to be employed full time by an organisation, and will not consider a lead applicant who only has an honorary contract or who has retired.

When the lead applicant does not have much experience in the field, usually because they are early on in their career, it is advisable to get at least 2 applicants who are experienced (see Section 7.5.6, page 110). However, this is not necessary when applying for training fellowships or doctoral degree grants.

The constitution and size of the Study Team will depend on the proposed study. Small studies, that will include only one or two centres, may require up to five people, while large multicentre studies which require input from several disciplines could have ten or more people. Some funding bodies specify a maximum limit to the number of co-investigators on a grant application. The Study Team (Box 2.1) usually has the following (where appropriate):

- Chief Investigator.
- At least one other health professional with expertise in the field of study.
- At least one person who will recruit subjects (often this person comes from the potentially largest centres).
- Statistician; this is mandatory for some funding bodies.
- Study co-ordinator.

At least one laboratory scientist.

Box 2.2 shows examples of research studies, and the roles of those who would be expected to form the Study Team. Most would also be named co-applicants on a grant application, except perhaps for the study co-ordinator, who might not be appointed until the grant is available. Most funding bodies will want to see evidence of direct input into the grant application from more than one health professional and, where appropriate, a statistician. Sometimes, the person who provided statistical input for the grant application is not the same as the study statistician who analyses the data and is only appointed once the application is successful.

It is useful for the Study Team to meet during the development of the grant application, either in person or by teleconference, to consider key

Box 2.1 Roles of people involved in a research study*

- *Centre Investigator*: A person who is responsible for conducting the study at a particular centre (or site), where research subjects (humans) are to be recruited or their records examined. Such individuals do not need to be named as co-applicants on the grant application, or be a member of the Study Team, but those from larger centres often are. If there are several investigators at a centre, one is usually named as the *principal investigator*. He/she is normally expected to have a full contract of employment.
- *Chief Investigator/Applicant (CI)*: A single named person responsible for the study design and conduct, and who acts as Chair of the Study Team. The CI is often the person who conceived the idea for the study or may be a key opinion leader in the area of work. He/she is named as the lead investigator on applications for grant funding, and regulatory and ethical approval when required. The CI often, but not always, works in the host institution. He/she is normally expected to have a full contract of employment.
- *Co-investigator (co-applicant)*: Someone with an area of expertise that is essential to the study. They are named on the grant application and should be part of the Study Team.
- *Collaborator or contributor*: Someone who is not part of the Study Team (because they do not have the same level of input) and does not recruit subjects, but has input into a specific issue on the design, conduct or analysis at some point. They could be, for example, a health economist, pathologist, consumer or patient representative, or expert scientist.
- *Co-ordinator*: Someone who is responsible for the day-to-day conduct of the study (usually in humans), for example setting up centres, dealing with queries, data management, recruiting subjects and (in multicentre studies) possibly overseeing staff within the other centres who deal with study subjects.
- *Laboratory or research assistant/technician*: A suitably qualified person with responsibility for developing or implementing a particular experimental or laboratory technique.
- *Sponsor*: A commercial company, institution or organisation which has ultimate responsibility for the initiation, management and financing of a research study, when it involves human subjects (usually clinical trials). The Sponsor must ensure that the study is conducted in accordance to any relevant national regulations and guidelines.
- *Statistician*: A suitably qualified person who is directly involved in the trial design, sample size estimation and statistical analysis of the study data.

*These are not fixed terms, but the descriptions are fairly standard. For example, health professionals who recruit subjects ('Centre Investigator' in the box) could be referred to as collaborators by some funding bodies; or a Chief Investigator is sometimes called the Principal Investigator.

Box 2.2 Examples of research studies and the types of people who could be part of the Study Team

Study description	Types of people/roles	Reason why the role is part of the Study Team
National clinical trial to compare two surgical approaches to treating oral cancer. The results would affect routine clinical practice.	Chief Investigator	Surgeon with many years of expertise in oral cancer.
	Two or three other surgeons	Need some agreement on the surgical approaches to be used in the trial.
	Statistician	Trial design and analysis.
	Trial co-ordinator	Daily management of the trial and recruitment.
	Pathologist	Central review of histological samples.
	Oncologist	Patients will often get chemotherapy after surgery, so need expertise in this therapy.
	Health economist	To help determine whether one approach is more cost-effective than the other.
International observational study to compare two different antenatal screening policies for Down's syndrome. The results would affect routine clinical practice.	Chief Investigator	Clinician with many years of expertise in antenatal screening.
	Three or four obstetricians	Need other experts in antenatal screening.
	Statistician	Study design and analysis.
	Study co-ordinator	Daily management of the study, and recruitment.
	Biochemist	Some of the screening tests involve a blood measurement.
	Ultrasonographer	One of the screening tests is an ultrasound examination of the foetus.
	Health economist	To help determine whether one approach is more cost-effective than the other.

Study description	Types of people/roles	Reason why the role is part of the Study Team
Survey of stroke recovery patients and their relatives, within a single hospital, to examine their experiences of the care received. The results could be used to improve the delivery of care at the hospital.	Chief Investigator	Clinician/psychologist with expertise in stroke.
	Two or three health professionals (psychologists and stroke clinicians)	People who would treat patients, or be able to design the questionnaires/ interviews for the study.
	Statistician	Study design and analysis.
	Research nurse	Study conduct, recruit patients and enter data onto database.
	Patient representative	Someone with personal experience who can help with the study design and interpretation of results.

design issues. Sometimes, the Chief Investigator will discuss the proposed project with the Study Team members separately, and collate the comments to produce a first draft of the application. Each revised version should be emailed to all the co-applicants, but it is important that they all review and approve the application before it is submitted.

2.1.1 Obtaining signatures of the co-applicants

It is often necessary for all co-investigators (co-applicants) to sign the application form. This provides evidence that the project is fully supported by the Study Team, and that it is likely to have been discussed properly. Sufficient time is needed to obtain all of the signatures; perhaps 2–4 weeks, depending on how many there are. Sometimes, it is acceptable not to have all the signatures on the same page, though researchers should check whether this is allowed with administrative staff at the funding body. For example, the lead (chief) applicant, host institution finance officer and Head of Department should sign on the same page, but the co-investigators could each sign a separate page and forward this onto the lead applicant. This is a quicker method of obtaining the necessary signatures than sending the same page to each individual in turn to sign.

2.2 Other investigators, collaborators and consultants

There may be people who are not part of the Study Team but who contribute to the project or grant application. Application forms may have separate sections for naming individuals who are on the Study Team (co-investigators or applicants) and those who are collaborators.

A *Centre Investigator* might be someone responsible for the study at a single recruiting centre (for studies of humans), or an individual responsible for providing advice on a specific activity in a laboratory experiment. This could be a senior health professional, and he/she may represent several others working at the centre when they are all involved in recruiting study subjects (i.e. a *Principal Investigator*). A principal investigator with recognised expertise and is based in a centre that is expected to accrue a significant proportion of all study subjects (perhaps >10%) might also be a co-applicant. For studies in which there will only be a few centres, such as early phase clinical trials, it may be appropriate to have an investigator from each centre on the Study Team. It is always useful to be able to list several named collaborators, particularly for large or complex studies, or those in uncommon disorders, because the study is highly unlikely to succeed without their support.

There could be other *collaborators* (*contributors*, *advisors* or *consultants*) who are not directly involved in designing or conducting the study, or recruiting subjects, but may still provide expertise for a specific part of the project or grant application. The following roles are sometimes included in this category, though in some cases they could be part of the Study Team and be a co-applicant if their input is judged to be great enough:

- Health economist
- Statistician
- Pathologist
- Health psychologist
- Patient or consumer representative
- Research nurse
- Expert on a particular laboratory method or technical equipment.

For example, studies on humans require a Participant Information Sheet to be given to all potential subjects, which could benefit from being reviewed by a study subject or research nurse involved in recruitment (see Section 5.2, page 73).

2.3 The host institution and Sponsor

In this book, the *host institution* is taken to be the organisation from which the proposed study will be conducted or co-ordinated. The Chief Investigator is usually employed there (Box 2.1). The host institution is named on the grant application, has approved the funding requested by the applicants, and if successful, will manage the grant, and employ staff to run the study. However, the Study Team will manage and have responsibility for the project itself.

When the study is to be based on human subjects (often for clinical trials), there is sometimes the concept of a named *Sponsor*. This is effectively the host institution, and it has ultimate responsibility for the study design and conduct, and should have oversight of the study across all the recruiting centres. Although these tasks are actually undertaken by the Study Team or investigators at recruiting centres, it is the responsibility of the Sponsor if anything goes wrong (e.g. a major error in the study protocol that leads to a subject being harmed). The Sponsor will therefore need to have adequate insurance and indemnity in place. A proposed human study is often expected to be registered with the Sponsor before the grant application is submitted. This is especially important for clinical trials of new and unlicensed drugs, or those in children or incapacitated adults. Clinical trials of investigational drugs almost always require a named Sponsor, by law in many countries. For all other trials and observational studies, applicants should check with their host institution whether the concept of a named Sponsor applies.

2.4 Commercial companies

A commercial company often provides free drugs or medical devices for an academic-led study, usually clinical trials, and occasionally may also cover part[2] or all of a grant to conduct the study. Although company representatives would not normally be part of the Study Team, they will expect to be involved throughout the study. This will include review and approval of the study protocol, any subsequent changes made to it and a regular update on the study while it is being conducted. Before the grant application is submitted, the study should be discussed with the company, which often has a proforma on which researchers provide the important details of the objectives and design. The company will need to provide a letter of support as part of the application if funded is sought elsewhere (see Section 5.5, page 76).

2.5 Oversight committees

It is good practice for a clinical trial of interventions in humans to have an independent oversight committee, and some large observational studies may also benefit from having one. This committee, chosen by the Study Team, is usually called an *Independent Data Monitoring Committee (IDMC)*, or *Data Monitoring and Ethics Committee (DMEC)*, and its purpose is to advise the Study Team. An IDMC usually consists of three to five people: health professionals, a statistician and other relevant experts with no direct connection to the trial.

---

[2] A governmental or charitable organisation could provide the rest of the grant.

They meet regularly to discuss the study, at least once a year in person or by teleconference, and are meant to provide an independent and unbiased review of the study during the recruitment and treatment periods, and sometimes also during the follow-up. Their main functions are to:

- Safeguard the interests of study subjects.
- Assess safety and adverse events.
- Identify poor recruitment.
- Monitor the overall conduct of the study, such as treatment compliance and missing data.
- Sometimes examine early data on efficacy.
- Suggest revisions to the study protocol when judged necessary.
- Recommend whether a study should be terminated early.

It is not commonplace to have an IDMC for early phase (I and II) trials because these tend to have a relatively small number of subjects and in any case should be closely monitored by the researchers. However, it is becoming increasingly common for phase II trials with new and unlicensed agents or randomised phase II studies to have an IDMC, in order to show the regulatory authority and Sponsor that safety and well-being are being monitored carefully and independently. Most phase III trials will an IDMC.

The grant application may have a section in which the applicants list the names of the IDMC, if already chosen. These would normally be professional colleagues of the Study Team but cannot be involved in the study, for example in the recruitment or management of the study participants. The IDMC members should be chosen on the basis of their expertise but also on their ability to provide sensible and constructive advice. If the Study Team is unsure about the names of the IDMC at the time of the grant application, it may be possible just to say that three to five people will be appointed with expertise in specific areas relevant to the study, then list these specialities.

For clinical trials on humans, an independent *Trial Steering Committee (TSC)*[3] is sometimes appointed in addition to an IDMC, and again there may be a section in the grant application to provide potential names. As with the IDMC, the TSC members will review features of the trial as it is being conducted, but they tend to focus on administrative and logistical problems such as poor recruitment, rather than safety or efficacy (the IDMC would send a report to the TSC as well as to the Study Team on these two aspects). While the IDMC advises the Study Team, the main purpose of a TSC is to

---

[3] Traditionally, a TSC was the Study Team (i.e. the people who designed and conducted the trial). However in some places this term is now used for an independent oversight committee.

advise the funding body, and it could have the authority to terminate a study early. The TSC members are often chosen by the Study Team, but in some instances the funding body may already have one established. A TSC may be responsible for having oversight of several studies.

Summary points

- Ensure that key people with the necessary expertise relevant to the proposed study are part of the Study Team, and have been involved in developing the application.
- Include many or all members of the Study Team as co-investigators on the grant application, when appropriate.
- The application should be sent to all co-applicants for final approval before being submitted.
- Identify collaborators who are likely to have an input into the project at some stage, which is not substantial.
- Have proper discussions with commercial companies who are expected to provide free materials for the study.
- The study idea and grant application should not be developed by only one or two people; make sure there is clear evidence of input from several people.
- Ensure that signatures are obtained from all the co-applicants.

Chapter 3 **Justification for the study**

Before developing the grant application it is worth ensuring that there is a need for the proposed study; there is likely to be sufficient interest from centres who would be expected to participate (when relevant); and that the results will be useful to others. Applicants should spend time obtaining this information, after discussion with members of the Study Team, and ensure that their knowledge is up-to-date.

3.1 Finding background information

Applicants should always first consult with their colleagues on whether their study is attractive and feasible, since even with the best intentions, some research ideas have major flaws that can be immediately spotted by an expert in the field. In addition to this, it is always worthwhile examining the medical literature and research study registers (Box 3.1) in order to:

- Succinctly describe the context of the proposed study (review articles can be particularly useful for this).
- Compile evidence as part of the justification for the proposed study.
- Determine whether studies similar to that proposed have already been done or are currently in progress elsewhere.

Finding information can be done using electronic databases of published journal articles, such as PUBMED or MEDLINE. Even an Internet search could yield useful information, but it is always best to obtain formal references to accompany a description justifying a new study. Applicants with a clinical trial should also look at international registers of past or ongoing trials (Box 3.1), which contain the names of the trials, their objectives, endpoints, eligibility criteria, target sample size, and start and expected end date

How to Write a Grant Application, 1st edition. © Allan Hackshaw. Published 2011 by Blackwell Publishing Ltd.

Box 3.1 Useful website addresses to find information associated with a proposed study

Electronic databases of abstracts of most published clinical articles:

- PUBMED: http://www.ncbi.nlm.nih.gov/pubmed
- MEDLINE: http://www.proquest. com/en-US/catalogs/databases/ detail/medline_ft.shtml
- EMBASE: http://www.embase.com/

Databases or registers of clinical trials:

- Cochrane library: http://www.thecochranelibrary.com/view/0/index.html
- ClinicalTrials.gov: http://clinicaltrials.gov/
- International Standard Randomised Controlled Trial Number (ISRCTN): http://www.controlled-trials.com/

---

of recruitment. It is now a requirement of many journals that the trial has been preregistered when they consider an article is submitted, and it is a legal requirement of trials sponsored in the United States. Some funding organisations require applicants to have checked for similar studies, and may request confirmation of this on the application form.

When searching for information using electronic databases, it is useful to be aware that researchers may use different spellings and different terminologies in their articles, and that medical journals have their own terminology house style. Otherwise it is possible that important studies may be missed. Examples are:

1 To find studies that have examined the association between an exposure and an outcome (e.g. maternal cigarette smoking and miscarriage of pregnancy); any of the following words could be used in a study abstract (in addition to 'smoking' and 'miscarriage' or 'spontaneous abortion'):
   - Risk factor(s).
   - Marker(s).
   - Prognostic factor(s).
   - Indicator.
   - Measure(s) of association.
2 Randomised clinical trials can be described in several ways:
   - Randomised or randomized.
   - Patients were randomly allocated to the trial interventions.
   - Patients were allocated to the trial interventions at random.

The use of wildcards (here, random$) should ensure that any of the above modifications of 'random' are picked up.

3.2 Previous evidence and similar research (why the study is needed now)

The justification for a study is often not well described in grant applications, yet it is an important feature. It should address some key questions (Box 3.2). Applicants should ensure that seminal and well-known published articles are referenced, when appropriate. With the Internet and international clinical trials registers, it is now easier to find out whether other researchers are currently conducting a similar study to the one proposed, and electronic databases of published articles can be used to find similar studies that have already been reported.

Box 3.2 Key considerations for justifying a proposed study

- Why is the study needed now (i.e. the context or background)?
- What supporting evidence is there for the study (i.e. biological plausibility, efficacy and safety of clinical trial interventions, and so on)?
- Will the study be feasible, and if so, is there any evidence of this?
- How will the results and conclusions be used?

Information found from the various sources mentioned in section 3.1 may be used to provide supporting or background evidence for the proposed study, such as the incidence of a disorder or the context of the problem to be addressed. There should be a clearly written section to show the funding body and its external reviewers why the proposed study is important, such as a common disorder with poor prognoses, or an uncommon disorder with few effective treatment options.

For example, if the study aims to compare two different antenatal screening methods for Down's syndrome, there should be a description of the prevalence of this disorder in pregnancy or at birth; the performance of current screening methods (e.g. detection and false-positive rates); and which new tests have recently come to light that are potentially more effective. Published references to this information should always be given where available. Another example could be a clinical trial to evaluate a new drug for advanced ovarian cancer. The applicants should mention the incidence, either as a rate per 1000, or the total number diagnosed per year in the relevant country; the median survival time using current standard therapies; and any prior evidence associated with the new treatment to be investigated in the proposed trial.

The existence of similar studies to the one proposed does not necessarily mean that applicants should not proceed. In fact, it is often good practice to replicate other research before there is a major change to health practice or policy, or scientific knowledge is updated. However, applicants need to bear in mind that the funding body may prefer to invest in something new or more novel. There are several other reasons why conducting a new study may still be justified. Previous studies could have:

- Had significant design flaws (e.g. inappropriate endpoints).
- Used out-of-date methodology.
- Had too few subjects to produce reliable conclusions.
- Been affected by significant bias or confounding.
- Been conducted in groups of people with different characteristics to the one proposed.

Applicants need to show convincingly that the proposed study will still contribute to knowledge if there have already been several similar studies on the same topic, otherwise the application probably has a low chance of being successfully funded. Systematic review articles can provide clearer answers to a research question than any single study on its own, but they could also be used to show that current evidence is lacking, and that a large new study is needed. An example is given in Box 3.3.

Box 3.3 Example of prior evidence (systematic review) being used to justify future studies (Hackshaw et al. 2007, Mallick et al. 2008)

- *Setting*: Patients with differentiated thyroid cancer are usually treated with a high dose of radioactive iodine after surgery (3.7 GBq). Patients, many of whom are young (i.e. <50 years) and with children, stay in hospital isolation for about 3 days. Radioactive iodine is also associated with side effects, including an increased risk of developing a new cancer in the future.

- *Proposed change in clinical practice*: To use a lower dose, 1.1 GBq, because patients should only be in hospital isolation for 1–2 days, there are fewer side effects, and their risk of a second future cancer is significantly reduced.

- *Prior evidence*: 53 observational studies (many involving retrospective analyses of patient medical records) and 6 randomised clinical trials, which compared the efficacy of low- versus high-dose radioactive iodine, were examined in a systematic review. However, the observational studies could be affected by bias and confounding, and all the comparisons of 1.1 versus 3.7 GBq from the clinical trials were based on a small number of patients (each <150 patients). Taken together the results were equivocal; some studies suggested that 1.1 GBq had a lower efficacy while others indicated that it had a similar effect to 3.7 GBq.

- *Recommendation*: Because of a lack of clear evidence, a large randomised national trial was designed and conducted in the United Kingdom to properly address the issue, with a target sample size of about 450 patients.

Ideally, the prior evidence should come from several good quality research articles,[1] and it can help if the results and conclusions are consistent with each other (though inconsistency could also be used to justify new work). Sometimes, the applicants themselves have conducted prior research, which is as yet unpublished. The grant application should provide a clear account of that study design, a summary of the key results and show how the conclusions have led to the proposed study. When there are several related published studies, a summary of them (e.g. design and key results) could be presented in a table and placed into an appendix (see Section 4.2, page 40). There should be an adequate number of references that are relevant to the proposed study, and this will vary according to the field of study and what published literature already exists. As a general rule, less than 10 references is probably too few and more than 100 is too many.

3.3 Biological plausibility

The background information, and evidence from similar previous studies, could also be used to develop the text on biological plausibility. This is essential for observational studies used to examine or identify risk factors, clinical trials of new interventions, or laboratory experiments which aim to test a certain hypothesis such as finding biomarkers for a disorder. The mechanisms should be outlined clearly in the application, with reference to published or unpublished work. The funding committee and external reviewers will want to see whether the mechanisms described are likely to support the main study hypotheses, and this will be partly influenced by the quality and strength of the references used by the applicants (see also Section 3.2).

Early phase I and II clinical trials of new interventions, such as investigational drugs, will often be supported by *in vitro* laboratory experiments. These may be published already, or in some instances they could come from internal studies conducted within pharmaceutical companies. Researchers proposing a large randomised phase III trial may be able to use positive results on efficacy from phase I and II studies (see Box 4.7, showing different phases), or sometimes from observational studies. Phase III trials tend to be based on several hundred or thousand subjects, may take several years to conduct and are expensive. Therefore, there should be good prior evidence that a new intervention is likely to be more effective than the control intervention (if looking for superiority), or that it is has a similar effect (if looking for equivalence or non-inferiority); see Box 4.8, page 53.

---

[1]These articles might also be used to discuss biological plausibility (Section 3.3).

3.4 Safety of new interventions in clinical trials

Applications associated with clinical trials should also include prior evidence on safety of new therapies, particularly for novel and unlicensed drugs or exposures, which are in early development. Applicants should describe the safety profile clearly (perhaps as a specific subsection), and ideally persuade the funding committee and external reviewers that the new intervention is likely to have acceptable side effects which should be outweighed by the potential clinical benefits (see also Section 4.9.3, page 67). As with efficacy, prior data on safety and toxicities of drugs or medical devices could come from the published literature or internal reports from pharmaceutical companies. A list of the main expected side effects (particularly the most serious or most common ones) should be given, along with an estimated proportion of subjects who could be affected by each event type.

Safety should be considered in relation to standard interventions currently being used, because the new intervention should not be associated with a much greater risk of adverse events. Sometimes, the new intervention is a standard therapy or exposure (such as radiotherapy) but used at a lower dose than usual, therefore safety could be used as part of the justification for the study.

3.5 Feasibility

The funding committee and its external reviewers will need to form a view on whether the proposed study is feasible. This generally means being convinced by the applicants that the study can be completed within a reasonable time frame and that the objectives can be addressed satisfactorily (see Section 7.5.5, page 109). Large, ambitious studies of humans, or laboratory experiments, tend to be the ones where feasibility may be an issue, and may therefore be more closely scrutinised.

For example, in a large cohort study or clinical trial, particularly if the disorder of interest is uncommon or the design is complex, it might be appropriate to first examine whether the target sample size is likely to be reached in the specified time frame. Applicants could indicate a realistic number of centres that may take part or a realistic monthly accrual rate; these should not be overestimated. A good approach is to undertake a simple survey of several potential centres (preferably some large ones) before the grant application is submitted, to find out if they might be interested in the proposed study, whether they have any major issues with the hypotheses or design, and to obtain an approximate number of subjects from each centre. Investigators at centres do not have to give a formal commitment to the study (see Section 5.4, page 76, other documents). The results of the survey could be used as supporting evidence in the application.

There are several reasons why a study may not be feasible, such as insufficient interest from potential participating centres, a lower than expected number of eligible subjects or insufficient interest by potential subjects. These reasons are themselves influenced by the complexity of the study, financial costs incurred by the participating centre or study subject, or the nature and frequency of examinations and tests during follow-up (e.g. invasive tests or too frequent examinations). If the funding committee or its external reviewers consider that feasibility is likely to be a major problem, they may raise this as a criticism of the study. It is usually better to pre-empt this by addressing the issue in the grant application, and provide some evidence of feasibility.

An assessment of feasibility could be an integral part of the project, to be made in the first 12–24 months of a study that would take several years to complete. It would involve determining whether the target sample size is likely to be reached, and if not, the study could terminate early, and no further funds are requested. This early stage evaluation is sometimes referred to as a *feasibility* or *pilot study*. Although it may or may not accurately reflect what will happen during the whole study, it often gives a good idea. There may not need to be a formal sample size calculation for this particular stage of the project, but it is worth being clear about which criteria need to be met before deciding whether the study should continue as planned. Feasibility studies are often based in a few centres first, rather than being opened up to many, because setting up studies can take several months so the researchers may choose to concentrate their resources. In the grant application, the applicants should list these centres, and provide letters of support (see Section 5.4, page 76).

Feasibility studies could raise issues that require investigation, for example, examining the proportion of eligible subjects approached who agree to participate (i.e. the *acceptance* or *uptake rate*), and if this is too low, what the likely reasons for this might be. For example, there could be randomised clinical trials where the test intervention is no treatment or less treatment, compared to the current standard therapy; a comparison of a simple and complex surgical operation; or short versus long duration of treatment. In any of these scenarios, trial subjects, when faced with both treatment options, may opt for one over the other, and hence decline to participate. It is worth discussing potential problems like these in the application.

Consider a cohort study requiring 3000 subjects to be recruited over 3 years. The feasibility study could be conducted to see whether a recruitment rate of 80–85 subjects per month is likely. The endpoint could be 'monthly accrual rate' assessed during months 6–12 after recruitment started, and ignoring the first 6 months when the centres have just been set up. If the accrual rate is low, ways could be found to encourage participation, perhaps by changing the wording of the Participant Information Sheet (see page 73) or finding

Box 3.4 An example of text addressing feasibility in a clinical trial

Sample size for the phase III trial:

The sample size estimate for the phase III trial is based on a 2-year overall survival rate in the control arm of 45%. We aim to detect a hazard ratio of 0.70 associated with the new intervention. Therefore, 270 patients per arm would be required (N = 540), with 80% power and two-sided 5% level of statistical significance, using a logrank test. To allow for a potential dropout rate of 5%, the trial would aim to recruit 570 patients in total.

Feasibility study (15 months, of which the first 3 months would be trial set-up)*:

Our target is to set up at least four centres initially, and each need to recruit an average of two patients per month during a 12-month period, to yield about 100 patients in total. If this can be achieved, the feasibility study would be regarded as successful. During the first 3 months of the feasibility study, our focus will be on setting up a minimum of four centres. However, we will also canvas interest from other centres and, where possible, activate them.

In order to achieve the additional recruitment needed in phase III, a further six centres of similar size would be required (or more if they have smaller patient numbers). Each of these would also be required to recruit two patients per month, on average. This could yield 580 patients: 10 centres × 24 patients each per year × 2 years = 480, plus the 100 from the feasibility study, allowing the sample size target of 570 to be reached. Alternatively, we would need to randomise a total of about 20 patients per month across all centres over 2 years.

*The feasibility study could be conducted with minimal financial support (e.g. part-time trial co-ordinator).

out whether recruiting centres are experiencing problems. Box 3.4 shows an example of text that could be used to describe feasibility, based on a phase III clinical trial.

3.6 What will the study contribute?

A vital part of the grant application is to describe how the results and conclusions of the proposed study might be used. This is done on the assumption that the study hypotheses are correct and the objectives will be met (in other words, the study is 'positive'). The application will be competing with others, and the potential contribution of the study will be a major factor in determining whether it is successfully funded (see also Section 7.5, pages 106–109).

There are several ways in which studies can be used, and this should be made explicit in the application. For example:

- Observational studies
  - to identify risk factors for disease or early death;
  - to gain a better understanding of people's behaviour and attitudes;
  - to change public health policy.
- Clinical trials of new interventions
  - to change clinical practice;
  - to justify and help design further trials (e.g. early phase I and II studies leading to phase III trials).
- Laboratory experiments
  - to advance scientific and biological knowledge;
  - to target treatments to certain subgroups of patients (e.g. those with certain biomarker or genetic profiles, as in translational research);
  - to identify new biomarkers, or genetic or imaging markers for disease or early death.

The originality or novelty of the study should also be addressed. When relevant, applicants should make clear whether the proposed study is:

- The first of its kind
  - the first to use a new therapy, or combination of new and existing therapies;
  - the first to use an existing therapy but in a new disease area;
  - the first to develop and implement a new laboratory technique;
  - the first to identify one or more new biological or genetic markers, or other factors, for a disorder or early death.
- Similar to previous studies but has major advantages, such as
  - it is the largest and will therefore provide more reliable data or a conclusive result;
  - it will be conducted in a different population;
  - it will use a more robust design (e.g. randomised trial, whereas previous evidence was based on observational studies);
  - it will use a novel design or experimental or laboratory method;
  - it will replicate other work to confirm previous results and conclusions.

3.7 Summary of the justification for a proposed study

After colleagues have been consulted, and information about related or similar previous research has been obtained, it should be possible to draft a summary for the grant application. There will usually be at least one specific section in the application form to discuss the justification of the study. It can be tempting to provide excessive information when there is extensive literature on the topic, or out of concern to cover as much as possible in the application to avoid missing an important aspect. However, it is important to concentrate on the key elements (Box 3.5) and avoid writing too much, because the application could otherwise appear to be unfocussed.

Box 3.5 Key points to consider when covering the justification for a proposed study

- What is the research topic to be addressed?
  - Define the disorder or problem in simple language.
- How important is it?
  - Prevalence, incidence or severity of the disorder; mortality estimate; survival time.
  - Current scientific knowledge.
  - How has the problem arisen in the past?
  - What has been the impact on health practice or society?
- Are there any limitations of previous similar research that could make their results or conclusions unreliable or not relevant?
  - Scientifically flawed.
  - Significantly affected by bias or confounding.
  - Studies have had too few subjects.
  - Studies were based on different subjects to the one proposed.
- Can the proposed study be successfully conducted?
  - There is sufficient interest from colleagues and potential participating centres.
  - There is prior evidence of safety (clinical trials of new interventions).
  - A *realistic* estimate of accrual (per month or per year) means that the study could be conducted within a reasonable time frame.
- What are the key attributes of the proposed study?
  - First of its kind.
  - Largest of its kind.
  - New or novel methods, techniques or interventions.
  - Will confirm results and conclusions from previous work.
- How will the results of the proposed study be used?
  - To plan and design further studies.
  - Change clinical practice or public health policy (either on its own or to replicate prior similar studies).
  - Provide new useful information to help health professionals in their work, including how they deal with patients or other individuals.
  - To increase understanding on biological, pharmacological, physiological or psychological mechanisms.

Summary points

- Ensure that the study (i) has scientific interest, (ii) is feasible and (iii) will contribute to current knowledge.
- Provide a list of good quality references that directly support the background to the study and biological plausibility.
- If the proposed study is similar to previous ones, explain why it is different or likely to be better.
- For studies of humans, try to conduct a simple survey of potential recruiting centres to ascertain interest and an approximate number of subjects per centre (i.e. evidence of feasibility).
- Explain clearly how the results and conclusions of the study are expected to be used.

Chapter 4 **Describing the study design**

Providing a clear and sufficiently detailed description of the proposed study is perhaps the most important part of the grant application. There are several key aspects that together constitute the 'study design' (Figure 4.1), and they should all be covered in the application.

4.1 Abstract

Most grant applications have a section towards the beginning in which applicants provide an *abstract* of the proposed study. This is a concise summary, which usually has a recommended word limit (200–400 words). It is often easier to draft the abstract after the justification (Chapter 3) and details of the study design (current chapter) have been specified. It is one of the most important sections of the application because it allows the funding committee and the external reviewers to obtain a quick overview of the study before reading and interpreting the details in subsequent sections. Sometimes, there are non-scientific members of the funding committee (who may, for example, represent patient or consumer groups), so it is important to use clear, non-technical language in the abstract where possible.[1] Many application forms suggest a structure to the abstract, but even if this were not done it is certainly worth using subheadings. Recommended headings, with an example from a clinical trial, are shown in Box 4.1. Each heading should have only one to three sentences or statements, and only the key points need

---

[1] For many laboratory experiments it is likely that the application would only be reviewed by experts in the field, so technical language may be acceptable if it is standard and commonplace.

How to Write a Grant Application, 1st edition. © Allan Hackshaw. Published 2011 by Blackwell Publishing Ltd.

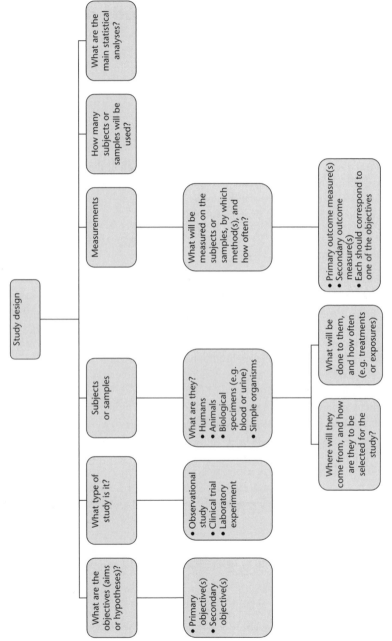

Figure 4.1 Specifications of the study design.

Box 4.1 Suggested subheadings for an abstract for a clinical trial (based on a published trial, Govaert et al. 1994); there are 204 words here

Heading	Example of text
Background	Influenza is an important public health problem for the elderly, which can lead to serious respiratory problems, hospitalisation and sometimes early death. Previous evidence of the flu vaccine has come only from observational studies, which could be affected by bias and confounding. We propose to conduct the first randomised trial.
Study design	Double-blind placebo-controlled multicentre randomised clinical trial of 1000 individuals.
Main eligibility	Individuals aged ≥60 years from a southern region in the Netherlands; no known previous history of heart or lung conditions, diabetes mellitus, chronic renal insufficiency or chronic staphylococcal infection.
Objectives	Primary: to determine the effectiveness of the flu vaccine in the elderly. Secondary: to examine the safety of the vaccine. To conduct a health economic assessment.
Interventions	Influenza vaccine or placebo (saline) injection given once. The vaccine will target four viral strains.
Outcome measures	Primary: incidence of influenza at 6 months determined by clinical assessment following symptoms. Secondary: incidence of influenza determined by serology and by self-assessment questionnaire; reported adverse events.
Assessments	Clinical assessment by a family physician using standardised criteria (International Classification of Health Problems in Primary Care). Health assessment questionnaire to be completed monthly. Blood sample at 6 months.
Trial duration	Recruitment 2 years; follow-up 1 year.

to be covered. Additional headings that may be appropriate for observational studies or laboratory experiments could be:
- Source of subjects
  - Where the subjects would be selected from (observational studies).
  - The number of cases and controls (case–control study), and the matching factors.
  - The animal species and strain, or key aspects of the biological samples used (laboratory experiments).

- Interventions or exposures (laboratory experiments)
  - Key features of the methodology, for example how it will be developed and implemented.
- Any translational research planned.
  - Which biological samples would be collected, and the biomarkers or genetic markers that might be examined.

The abstract should be considered by, and have input from, as many Study Team members as possible, and may need to go through several revisions before the text is sufficiently polished. The usual required text font size is often 12, but if the abstract does not fit onto a single page (often within a bordered section) it might be possible to reduce the font size, but less than size 10 could make the text appear too small and cramped.

It is worth having a simple flow diagram for studies of humans as illustrated in Figure 4.2 (though some laboratory experiments may also benefit from this). It should show the *key* design features at a glance, that is:

(A)

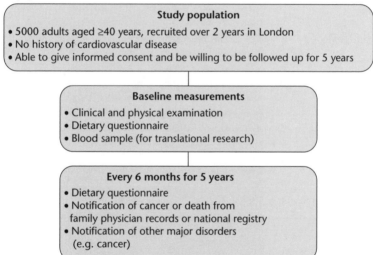

Figure 4.2 Flow diagrams for (A) a hypothetical cohort study examining the association between diet and heart disease, and (B) a randomised clinical trial in treating thyroid cancer comparing radioiodine ablation with no ablation (primary endpoint is recurrence-free survival).

(B)

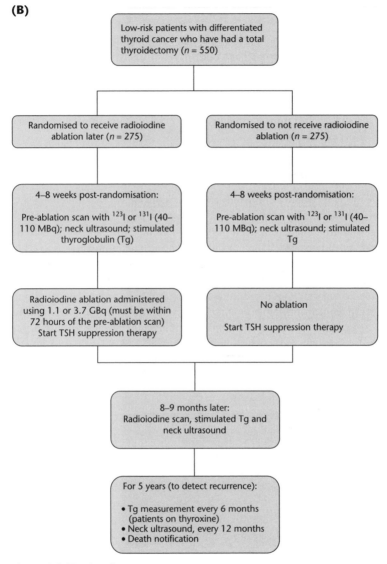

Figure 4.2 (*Continued*)

- The main (two or three) eligibility criteria, which largely define the study population.
- What happens to the subjects at the start of the study (e.g. baseline assessments or interventions). For a randomised clinical trial, indicate when the randomisation occurs.
- What happens during the study (e.g. follow-up assessments).

If there is an embedded translational research study, this could also be indicated on the diagram. For example, if a biomarker or imaging marker is used to select eligible subjects.

4.2 Appendices

The sections below cover details about the study design that are expected to be provided in the grant application. However, there will usually be a limit to the amount of text that can be provided on the form, so applicants could add appendices, which are not included in the maximum allowed word or page count. These should not be used to overload the funding committee with as much information as possible. Appendices should be few in number, concise and only contain additional necessary details that are likely to interest the funding committee or external reviewers. For example, there could be details about a previously unpublished study that is being used as supporting evidence for the proposed study, a summary of the key results and conclusions from several published similar studies, or additional technical details about a laboratory experiment.

4.3 Study objectives and outcome measures

The study *objectives* (*aims* or *hypotheses*) should be clear, easy to read and written in non-technical language if possible, particularly when the funding committee or its external reviewers include non-scientific people, such as patient representatives. There are several categories of objectives (see Section 1.1, page 2).

Applicants should aim to describe each objective with one concise sentence; if much longer, this could indicate that the objective is unrealistic or the Study Team is unfocussed. Objectives of the study should not be confused with the *endpoints* (*outcome measures*). An endpoint is the quantitative measure that is used to address the objective. Box 4.2 shows examples of these. Common criticisms are when an inappropriate endpoint is used as the primary outcome measure, or important endpoints are not included at all. This is why it is important for the project to be discussed fully by the Study Team.

Box 4.2 Examples of objectives and corresponding outcome measures

Objective	Outcome measure or endpoint
To determine the effectiveness of statin therapy in people with no history of heart disease.	Mean serum cholesterol level.
To determine the effectiveness of statin therapy in people with a history of heart disease.	The proportion of people who have a second heart attack (incidence).
To determine whether new Therapy A for asthma has a similar effect to standard therapy.	The proportion of patients who suffer a severe asthma exacerbation.
To show whether Test A is better than Test B in identifying pregnant women carrying a Down's syndrome foetus.	• The proportion of women with a Down's syndrome pregnancy identified as test-positive (detection rate). • The proportion of women without a Down's syndrome pregnancy identified as test-positive (false-positive rate).
To examine the relationship between blood pressure and age.	Blood pressure and age obtained for every study subject.
To evaluate the effectiveness of chemotherapy in treating lung cancer.	Overall survival: the time from randomisation until death from any cause or date last seen alive.
To examine how developmental Vaccines C, D and E affect bacteria X.	The proportion of bacteria in each sample that dies when exposed to a vaccine.
To find a safe dose of a new drug in rodents before it is tested on humans.	The dose of drug that is associated with death in 10% of the rodents.

Each objective (hypothesis) should be associated with an outcome measure. Ideally there should be one, perhaps two, *main* or *primary objectives*. If there are several main objectives or hypotheses, these should be clearly justified. Applicants need to ensure that the study they are proposing is not overly complex or ambitious, and that the project can be completed in a reasonable time frame. The primary objectives and corresponding outcome measures are those that will be used to determine what happens after the study has finished and been reported. For example, they may be used to change clinical practice, develop public health policy, or advance scientific knowledge. *Secondary objectives* are usually used to provide additional information.

Box 4.3 is an example of a new drug for breast cancer to be given before surgery. If the new treatment has a clear benefit on overall survival (the primary endpoint), then it is likely to be adopted into routine clinical practice. However, if there is little or no effect on survival and only tumour response is improved, this is unlikely to persuade policy makers to use it, because tumour shrinkage does not necessarily lead to a lower risk of death. Instead, it just provides some useful information about the biological action of the drug. It is not good practice to change a secondary endpoint to a primary one after the results have been examined and there is no clear effect on the original primary endpoint.

Box 4.3 Possible primary and secondary objectives for a clinical trial of pre-operative New Drug A for breast cancer. The corresponding endpoint is indicated in each objective

Primary
- To evaluate the effectiveness of New Drug A in treating early breast cancer, in relation to overall survival.

Secondary
- To evaluate whether New Drug A has an effect on tumour response (i.e. tumour shrinkage).
- To evaluate whether New Drug A reduces the chance of cancer recurrence.
- To determine the safety (toxicity profile) of New Drug A.
- To determine whether New Drug A improves health-related quality of life.

Having well-defined objectives and corresponding clear outcome measures make it easier to:
- Decide what data to collect and how.
- Analyse the data.
- Interpret the results.
- Write the final report or paper for publication in a journal.

4.3.1 Surrogate outcome measures
In clinical trials of humans (and some laboratory animal experiments), there is the concept of a *true* or *surrogate* outcome measure for several disorders

(FDA 2007, Katz 2004, Temple 1999). A true endpoint usually has an obvious and direct clinical relevance to the study subjects, for example, whether they

- Live or die.
- Develop a disorder or not.

Surrogate endpoints are measures that do not often have an obvious impact that subjects are able to identify easily. Surrogate markers can be a blood measurement or the results of an imaging scan which usually lie along the same disease causal pathway as the true endpoint. For example, the incidence of a heart attack is a true endpoint in a trial of statin therapy and the prevention of coronary heart disease, but serum cholesterol is an accepted surrogate endpoint. A claim in benefit for a new drug need only come from a randomised trial in which cholesterol levels have been significantly reduced. Surrogate and true endpoints should be closely correlated: a change in the surrogate endpoint now is likely to produce a change in a true endpoint later.

Surrogate measures are attractive because there are usually more events than a true endpoint, and they occur in a shorter space of time. They are therefore commonly used in early phase clinical trials (phase I and II; see pages 50–52). Surrogate endpoints should not be specified as the primary outcome measure for phase III trials or large observational studies (when relevant) unless their value has already been established. However, there are occasions when a surrogate endpoint might be the only feasible way of evaluating a new intervention in a confirmatory phase III trial, for example when dealing with rare disorders or events, so their use should be properly justified in the grant application when specified as the primary outcome measure. It is acceptable to use surrogate endpoints as secondary outcome measures.

4.3.2 Quality control and central reviews

Several studies involve the collection and analysis of markers from biological samples, imaging scans, or pathology reports, as part of the evaluation of the main study endpoint(s). Alternatively, they could be used to select eligible subjects, or assign interventions or exposures to different subgroups defined by levels of a bio- or imaging marker. Where appropriate (or feasible), it is often worthwhile describing quality control mechanisms in the grant application, such as standardised central assessments or reviews, in order to improve the accuracy or precision of the results, and reduce variability. For example, non-standard or new biochemical markers could be measured in a central laboratory, and imaging scans and pathology reports could benefit from central review by 2–3 appropriate experts (who are perhaps blinded to any clinical outcomes of the study subject to avoid bias).

4.4 Types of studies

There are two broad types of study designs (*observational* and *experimental*), and the most appropriate should be used for addressing the objectives (Box 4.4). Either of these types of studies can be included in a *systematic review*. Detailed descriptions of the different types of studies can be obtained from books or articles such as those listed in the references on pages 120–121, but relevant attributes for the grant application are covered in Sections 4.5–4.7.

Box 4.4 Types of studies

Observational studies – the study subjects are observed in their natural conditions, and there is no intention to intervene:

- Qualitative research studies.
- Cross-sectional studies.
- Audits of patient data.
- Case–control (retrospective) studies.
- Cohort (prospective) studies.

Experimental studies – some or all study subjects are exposed to or treated with a substance or intervention that they would not normally receive:

- Clinical trials of humans.
- Laboratory experiments.

Systematic reviews (including meta-analysis) – the aim is to identify all published and unpublished studies in a particular area and combine their results. This is usually done for human studies:

- Clinical trials.
- Cohort and case–control studies.

It is important to be clear about which type of study would be considered by a particular funding organisation, or a particular subcommittee of the organisation, and this can be checked in the terms and conditions available on their website or documentation on request. A significant proportion of grants are only available for experimental studies such as laboratory experiments and clinical trials in humans. In many situations, it is also worth justifying the choice of study design, and explain why alternatives are less good or inappropriate.

4.5 Observational studies in humans

Observational studies are those in which usual practice is observed and measured. Data may be collected using questionnaires or face-to-face interviews with people, by non-participant observation, or by obtaining data from hospital or primary care records, or regional or national registries and datasets. The accuracy and completeness of data is an important consideration in observational studies, and will vary according to whether the data is self-reported by the study subject, comes from medical records, or direct diagnosis from a clinician.

Qualitative research studies (Pope & Mays 2006) tend to have relatively few subjects (say <50), and are usually based on observation or interviews with open-ended questions that allow the interviewer to probe further where appropriate. Qualitative research can be used in developing the design of quantitative studies, or their measurement instruments (e.g. questionnaires). In other situations, they are used to elicit opinions, for example what people think of a certain health service they have received, or why they do not want to accept a type of treatment.

Cross-sectional studies (Rothman 2002, Silman & MacFarlane 2002) can be used when the study objective is one of enquiry, monitoring or surveillance, for example, describing the characteristics or attitudes of a group of people on a range of topics. They are sometimes used to examine the association between risk factors and a disorder. Such studies tend to be funded when based on many subjects and use validated questionnaires. Sometimes, validated questionnaires are unavailable or inappropriate for the proposed study, so new questionnaires need to be specially designed. In this situation, applicants should describe the development process and how they will evaluate the validity of the new questionnaire.

Audits of patient data involve extracting data already contained in medical notes of past patients in hospitals or general practice, and using this information to examine interventions or risk factors for disease or early death. They are sometimes used as an alternative to other observational studies or clinical trials, but applicants need to be aware of their limitations, such as selection bias.

Case–control and *cohort studies* (Rothman 2002, Silman & MacFarlane 2002) are commonly used to examine risk factors for or causes of a disorder or early death, and occasionally interventions to prevent or treat disease (MacMahon & Collins 2001). Case–control studies take people with and without the disorder in a particular time period,[2] and compare the proportions who were or were not exposed in the past by asking them about their previous habits or lifestyle characteristics, or measure some biochemical or genetic marker. Prospective cohort studies are based on people without the disorder and researchers ascertain whether they are

---

[2] Or have died or not died.

or have been exposed to a factor of interest at baseline; other information is also collected at the same time. The subjects are then followed up over time, often several years, and the proportions who develop the disorder of interest are compared between those who were or were not exposed to the factor at baseline. There are also (i) *retrospective cohort studies*, in which baseline measurements and the follow-up period have both occurred already in the past, and the study involves collecting data from medical records or regional or national datasets, and (ii) *nested case–control studies*, in which a sample of cases and matched controls are selected from a cohort study.

Choosing between a case–control or cohort study depends on several considerations, including:

- How difficult it is to obtain the study participants (e.g. uncommon disorders or rare events).
- Whether the results are likely to be affected by bias and confounding, and to what extent.
- Financial costs.
- Study duration.

Cohort studies are generally regarded as providing more reliable evidence than case–control studies because they are less affected by recall bias (people with a disorder are more likely to recall past habits accurately than people without the disorder) or selection bias. However, cohort studies can take several years to conduct and therefore are often expensive. When the disorder of interest is uncommon or where the study duration needs to be limited, case–control studies are more appropriate because many more affected individuals can be obtained than with a cohort study, in a reasonable timeframe. Cohort studies are often used when the disorder is fairly common (e.g. an annual incidence of at least 10%). Certain study designs are better than others at minimising bias (e.g. recall bias, selection bias, information bias, observer bias and non-response bias). It is difficult, if not impossible, to allow for bias at the end of a study, so it is important that applicants address this in the design.

Important confounding factors can be allowed for in the design stage of a matched case–control study but not a cohort study (in which confounders are incorporated in the statistical analysis at the end of the study). Applicants could provide some justification for the choice of potential confounders, and some comment on the ability to measure them in a standard, accurate or complete way (e.g. ethnicity is often incomplete in questionnaires, and alcohol intake is often inaccurate).

Furthermore, it is only possible to estimate incidence (or risk) from cohort studies, not case–control studies.

4.5.1 Study design and conduct

Box 4.5 shows the main areas to cover when describing how an observational study is to be conducted. Selecting the subjects is an important consideration, particularly controls in case–control studies, which could come from the general population, hospital patients or relatives of the cases.

Box 4.5 Specific areas of study design to cover when describing observational studies

Section	What to cover (when appropriate)
Study subjects	• Specification of where exactly the subjects will come from, that is the sampling frame for all subjects. • A list of the inclusion and exclusion criteria. • How will subjects be selected from the sampling frame (e.g. random sampling, random digit telephone dialling, or consecutive cases and controls)? • Clear definition of cases and controls (case–control study).

	• Where will the controls come from?
	  • General population
	  • Hospital patients
	  • Primary, secondary or community care patients
	  • Relatives of cases.
	• Whether controls will be matched to cases and, if so, specify the matching factors (case–control study only).

Recruitment and follow-up	• The time period used to identify the subjects. • Length of recruitment and follow-up (cohort studies) • How far back into the past will they be asked to recall details about their lifestyle and habits (case–control studies)?
Assessments of subjects; collecting data	• A detailed description of how subjects will be assessed: • Method of data collection, e.g. face-to-face interviews, self-completed questionnaires, data from patient records, or use of regional or national datasets or registries

(Continued)

Box 4.5 (Continued)

- Whether there will be any additional assessments such as clinical or imaging examinations, or tests in blood, urine or saliva
  - Who will make the assessments?
  - The frequency of each assessment
- Any collection of biological samples (e.g. blood, urine) for central storage and future analyses, or use in the main study.
- How will important potential confounding factors be measured?
- How will potential biases be minimised?
- Details of how diagnoses of disorders will be made.
- How long will subjects be in the study (cohort study)?
- Whether there is any translational research, and the proposed biomarkers?

A *sampling frame* is usually needed and should be clearly defined. It can take many forms depending on the study, and examples are given in Box 4.6. Subjects are identified from the sampling frame and they may then be checked against the *eligibility criteria* before being included in the study. A simple eligibility criteria list for looking at the association between smoking and cancer could be:

- Inclusion criteria
  - Aged 18–80 years
  - Current or never-smokers
  - Able to give informed consent.
- Exclusion criteria
  - Currently being treated for cancer
  - Previous history of cancer
  - Occupational exposures known to be associated with high risk of cancer.

Having well defined eligibility criteria makes it easier for the funding committee and the external reviewers to see who exactly would be included in the study. Sometimes it is worth justifying the major criteria, for example, whether older people are to be excluded and, if so, why.

Box 4.6 Examples of sampling frames

Study and objective	Sampling frame	Method for selecting subjects from the sampling frame
Cross-sectional survey to estimate the prevalence of alcohol use and smoking among dental under-graduate students.	Register of all dental students in one dental school in the United Kingdom in 1998.	All students on the register.
Case–control study to examine the association between birth defects and maternal smoking.	Cases (babies with a birth defect) to be selected from a national birth defects registry (e.g. United Kingdom). Controls (unaffected babies) to be selected from all women who gave birth in a particular geographical region.	Cases: all affected babies on the national registry 1995–2005. Controls: random selection of unaffected babies born 1995–2000, matched for maternal age and birth year.
Cohort study to examine the association between exercise and the risk of heart disease.	All patients aged over 40 years who are registered with a physician in a particular geographical region.	5000 to be selected at random.

4.6 Clinical trials in humans

Clinical trials in humans are specifically designed to intervene in an individual's life, and then evaluate some health-related outcome with one or more of the following objectives:

- To diagnose or detect disease.
- To treat an existing disorder.
- To prevent disease or early death.
- To change behaviour, habits or other lifestyle factors.

(See Hackshaw 2009, page 120, for a comprehensive overview of clinical trials in humans, including objectives, choosing outcome measures and designs.)

Any administered drug or micronutrient that is examined in a clinical trial with the specific purpose of treating, preventing or diagnosing disease is usually referred to as an *Investigational Medicinal Product (IMP)* or *Investigational New Drug (IND)*.[3] People who take part in a trial can be referred to as 'subjects' or 'participants' (if they are healthy individuals), or 'patients' (if they are already ill).

Applicants should be aware of any regulations or guidelines that apply to clinical trials:

- The principles of Good Clinical Practice (www.ich.org); a set of international guidelines that recommend how trials should be set up and conducted, and study subjects managed.
- National regulations, such as the EU Clinical Trials Directive (European countries), or the Food and Drug Administration (FDA) regulations (United States).

4.6.1 Types of clinical trials (humans)

Most clinical trials on humans are generally categorised into three phases (I, II and III), and the phase used in the proposed study could be made clear in the application (Box 4.7).

Phase I trials

There are various designs for phase I trials (3+3, continuous reassessment and Bayesian methods), and applicants should specify which they intend to use. Many phase I studies involve identifying and acting on a *dose-limiting toxicity (DLT)*; an adverse event judged to be caused by the trial treatment, and may be severe enough to warrant other treatment and/or the trial treatment to stop. Applicants should define what they consider to be a DLT in the application. Dose-escalation studies also involve finding the maximum tolerated dose (MTD), which would be used in later trials, and choosing the MTD should be described.

---

[3] IMP in the European Union, and IND in the United States and Japan.

Box 4.7 General categorisation of clinical trials

Phase I
- First time a new drug or regimen is tested on humans; subsequent phase I trials could examine how best to administer the new treatment (e.g. time of day, with or without food).
- Sometimes called dose-finding or dose-escalation studies, when several drug doses are to be examined.
- Could be based on healthy volunteers or patients who are already ill.
- Few participants (e.g. <30).
- Primary aims are to find a dose with an acceptable level of safety (i.e. the maximum tolerated dose), or examine the biological and pharmacological effects.

Phase II
- Single-arm studies: all subjects given the new intervention.
- Randomised studies: there could be at least one new intervention to choose from (i.e. which would be investigated further), with or without a control group.
- Not too large, say 30–70 people per group.
- Surrogate outcomes measures are often the primary endpoint.
- Aim is to obtain a *preliminary* estimate of the effectiveness of a new intervention (before embarking on a larger, and more expensive, confirmatory trial).
- Results are often used to design a subsequent phase III trial.

Phase I/II
- A dose-finding phase I study is first conducted, from which the chosen dose is used in a subsequent phase II study.
- Reduces the time taken to obtain an initial evaluation of an intervention, because it avoids having to set up and conduct two separate studies.

Phase III
- Must be randomised and with a comparison (control) group which is given a standard therapy, placebo or no intervention.
- Relatively large (usually several hundred or thousand people).
- Aim is to provide a *definitive* answer on whether a new intervention is better than that administered to the control group, or is similarly effective but there are other advantages.
- Results should be precise and robust enough to persuade health professionals to change practice.

Phase II trials

There are various types of phase II trials from single-arm studies (one- or two- stage designs) to randomised studies with several new interventions to examine. When there are several new therapies, applicants should specify how they intend to choose which one(s) would be investigated further, for example, in a subsequent phase III trial.

Randomised phase II studies with a control group are becoming more common. The controls are given standard therapy, placebo or no intervention, whichever is appropriate. Traditionally, results from single-arm phase II trials were used with information from historical controls (published data from past patients) to design a phase III trial, primarily to estimate the possible treatment effect and sample size. However, one of the problems with using older data is that they may not be representative of subjects currently seen in practice, and this in turn affects the sample size for the phase III study. Therefore, using concurrent controls is best, and there is now a general preference for *randomised controlled phase II trials*. Applicants should aim to use these where possible or feasible, either with 1:1 randomisation or 2:1 (i.e. half as many controls as the new intervention, if recruitment might be an issue). However, single-arm phase II studies should be acceptable when, for example, (i) the target group is a rare disorder or subgroup, (ii) for proof-of-concept trials of newly developed drugs[4] or (iii) if there is good recent data for historical controls. Any of these would otherwise take too long if a randomised controlled phase II study were used.

If a phase II trial is to be based on the combination of a new drug plus standard therapy, but there is only prior safety evidence of the drug when used on its own, it might be worth having a preceding *'run-in' phase I study*, for example, of 6–12 patients and one or two dose levels. This is to ensure that there is no undue harm when subjects take the combination at the specified dose of the new drug, for example, due to an unexpected interaction. This would be part of the same design (and funding application), and it demonstrates to the funding committee and external reviewers that safety will be considered carefully.

Phase III trials

All phase III trials are randomised, with a control group, and the effects of confounding and most biases are minimised by design. There

---

[4]A small initial single-arm phase II study used to see if the new drug has some beneficial effect on an important clinical outcome. Larger phase II studies, including those with a control arm, could follow if the proof-of-concept study is positive.

are three categories of objectives which a phase III trial may seek to demonstrate, and this should be specified in the application (Box 4.8). For equivalence or non-inferiority studies, applicants should describe why the new intervention would be preferable to standard practice, for example whether it is expected to be safer, less expensive or more easily administered. This should be included in the justification for the study (see Section 3.4, page 29).

Box 4.8 Phase III trial objectives

	Comparing two interventions, A and B
Objective to be demonstrator	(B could be the standard treatment, placebo or no intervention)
Superiority	A is more effective than B
Equivalence	A has a similar effect to B
Non-inferiority	A is not less effective than B (i.e. it could have a similar effect or be more effective)

'Effect' or 'effective' can be associated with any primary trial endpoint, such as death, or occurrence or recurrence of a disorder

---

It should be clearly specified whether the subjects or the research team (i.e. the Study Team and any staff within centres involved in recruiting, treating or managing the trial subjects) know which intervention will be allocated (*single* or *double blinding*), and if a placebo will be used. The placebo effect is another bias that can be minimised by design, and applicants should consider a dummy intervention when feasible, possible or acceptable. The application should also indicate whether there are independent groups of subjects where each subject receives only one intervention (*parallel groups*; a standard two-arm trial), or that each subject will receive all the trial interventions (*crossover trial*).

Crossover trials could be affected by a *residual* (*carryover*) *effect*, in which the first treatment influences the response to the second treatment, making it difficult to distinguish the individual effects reliably. This could be overcome by having a sufficiently long *washout period* – a time between the two trial treatments when neither is given. This should be made clear in the application, and the length of time depends on the aetiology of the disorder of interest and the pharmacological properties of the treatments; some drugs may require only a few days, others a few weeks. If there is uncertainty over the length of washout period or the carryover effect, it may be preferable to use a standard two-arm trial.

Phase II/III trials
Traditionally, researchers would conduct a phase II trial first, and if the results were positive, they would set up and conduct a completely separate phase III trial afterwards. Data from trial subjects in the phase II trial would not be used in phase III. This can significantly increase the time taken to evaluate a new intervention by 2 or more years, because of the need to set up separate trials (i.e. two applications for ethics, institutional and national regulatory approvals, and a completely different group of trial subjects). A more efficient and cost-effective approach is to have a randomised controlled phase II trial, which can lead directly into phase III (as long as the eligibility criteria were very similar), which avoids having two separate groups of trial subjects. The phase II assessment involves determining whether the new intervention is potentially effective, and if not, no further subjects are recruited. This could be done using the same primary endpoint as the phase III assessment, or a surrogate marker for it. If the trial does continue to phase III, a larger number of subjects are recruited, but the primary results of the phase II stage should not be published. A phase II/III study can be particularly useful for uncommon disorders.

If this design is proposed, applicants should describe the conditions for moving to phase III (e.g. the target effect size[5], or p-value cut-off), and state who will review the data from the phase II stage (this is best done by an IDMC; the study investigators should not see the results). A possible alternative to a phase II/III design is to have a phase III trial directly but with an early assessment for superiority or futility (see Section 4.9.2, page 65). A major difference is that the funding organisation may only need to initially commit money for the phase II stage (with a II/III design), instead of the whole trial (phase III).

4.6.2 Specifying the objectives according to the phase of trial
The wording of the objectives should be consistent with the phase of trial. Phase I studies can be easy to describe because they focus mainly on safety or pharmacological effects. Efficacy is usually the primary objective of phase II and III trials. However, phase II trials are not designed to provide definitive evidence on efficacy, because they often do not have a comparison (or control) group, the sample size is always significantly smaller than that for a corresponding phase III trial, or the primary endpoint is a surrogate outcome. With this in mind, the objectives of phase II trials should

---

[5] See section 4.9 for definition.

be phrased using words such as 'to examine' or 'to investigate', to avoid suggesting that the trial results will show conclusively whether the new intervention works or not (Box 4.9). For phase III trials, stronger words such as 'to evaluate', 'to show' or 'to determine' are perhaps more appropriate.

4.6.3 Eligibility criteria

All clinical trials should have an *eligibility list*, containing the *inclusion* and *exclusion criteria*, which describes how subjects will be selected for the study. There may be a specific section for this in the application form. Each study will have its own criteria depending on the objectives. For example, many clinical trials typically include an age range, no serious co-morbid conditions, the ability to obtain consent, and that subjects have not previously taken the

---

Box 4.9 Examples of descriptions of objectives and endpoints according to phase of clinical trial

Phase of trial	Objective	Outcome measure (endpoint)
I	To determine the maximum tolerated dose of a new therapy for advanced colorectal cancer.	The number of patients who suffer a dose-limiting toxicity.
II	To investigate Drug A in patients with Parkinson's disease.	The proportion of patients in whom the disorder progresses after 1 year.
II	To examine the effect of Therapy B for lung cancer.	The proportion of patients who have a partial or complete tumour response at the end of treatment (i.e. tumour shrinkage).
III	To evaluate the effectiveness of a flu vaccine in the elderly.	The proportion of people who develop flu within 6 months (incidence).
III	To determine the effectiveness of statin therapy in people without a history of heart disease.	Mean serum cholesterol level 12 months later.
III	To show whether a new therapy for asthma has a similar effect as standard treatment.	The proportion of patients who suffer a severe asthma exacerbation during 1 year.

trial treatment. The inclusion and exclusion criteria should have unambiguous definitions so that the funding committee and the external reviewers can see exactly which subjects would be studied.

4.6.4 Study design and conduct

Box 4.10 shows the main areas to cover when describing how a clinical trial is to be conducted. When using a randomised trial, it is important that the schedule of follow-up assessments is as similar as possible between the intervention groups, in order to minimise bias, otherwise subjects in one group may tend to be seen more often than in the other group (or using different assessment methods), and this could over- or under-estimate the magnitude of the outcome measures.

Box 4.10 Specific areas of study design to cover when describing clinical trials

Section heading	What to cover (when appropriate)

Trial Design	• Main features of the trial
	  • Phase I, II or III (or I/II, II/III)
	  • Randomised or single arm
	  • Single or double blind (specify the placebo intervention).
	• If randomised, the method of allocation (i.e. simple, stratified or minimisation), and any stratification factors.

Study subjects	• Where will subjects be recruited from? • A list of the inclusion and exclusion criteria.

Interventions	• A clear description of what the trial interventions are, including:
	  • How they will be administered (e.g. oral, topical, injection, inhaled, change in behaviour or diet)
	  • The dose
	  • Frequency and duration of treatment.
	• Where relevant, justify the chosen doses and treatment frequency.
	• If subjects suffer an adverse event, specify whether the trial treatment stops or the dose is reduced (and then specify the dose reduction schedule).
	• Any other treatments to be given at the same time.
	• If free drug or medical devices are supplied, for example, by a pharmaceutical company, this should be stated.

Section heading	What to cover (when appropriate)
Recruitment and follow-up	• The length of the recruitment and follow-up periods (when added together they represent the total length of the trial).
	• Many trials will specify an 'active' phase, which ends when the last patient has completed the last protocol visit and the trial treatment is stopped. The follow-up phase begins after this.
	• The end of trial could be when the last subject has finished treatment or the results of the study are available (after sufficient follow-up), whichever occurs first. Alternatively, it could be a fixed time period after the last subject has been recruited (e.g. 12 months later).
Assessments of subjects; collecting data	• A detailed description of how subjects will be assessed:
	• What will happen at each visit (e.g. clinical examinations, biochemical tests, imaging tests, or questionnaire)
	• The frequency of each assessment (i.e. how often)
	• Any collection of biological samples (e.g. blood, urine, tissue) for central storage and future analyses, or use in the main trial?
	• How long subjects will be in the trial?
	• Whether there is any translational research and the proposed biomarkers.
Safety monitoring	• A list of known adverse reactions associated with the trial treatments.
	• Describe procedures for identifying and monitoring adverse events (e.g. stopping guidelines, see section 4.9.3, page 67).

4.7 Laboratory experiments

There is a large variety of laboratory experiments that can involve animals, biological samples (specimens) from humans or animals, or simple organisms such as viruses and bacteria, and therefore a wide range of study designs. Those based on animals or simple organisms are sometimes similar to clinical trials on humans, in that they involve the administration of an intervention or exposure, and interest is in how they respond. Animal experiments are carefully regulated in most countries. Applicants should justify why the study requires the specified species, and ensure that the minimum number of animals is used. Applicants may also need to be aware of any national or international guidelines, such as Good Manufacturing Practice (GMP), Good Laboratory Practice (GLP) or Good Clinical Practice for Clinical Laboratories that could be relevant to their research (see references for FDA Good Manufacturing Practice, and Medicines and Healthcare products Regulatory Agency (MHRA), GMP and GLP, page 120).

Many experiments involve the application of standard laboratory techniques to new areas of research, or the development of new methods. This should be described clearly in the application, with sufficient detail to enable the funding committee and external reviewers to see what is involved, and to comment on the methodology and any likely major difficulties. Applicants should list all the *key* reagents, assays, materials or equipment necessary for the experiment, indicating which are standard, and perhaps also the manufacturers (especially if items will be provided for free). It might also be useful to indicate where potential major problems may arise.

Describing the study hypotheses clearly is important to facilitate an understanding of how the different stages of an experiment could be used to address each hypothesis. The experiment could involve the development of new techniques; finding new biomarkers, protein markers, gene profiles, or gene expressions; or examining how levels of a measurement change over time, perhaps with and without the administration of different exposures. There may also be translational research projects (see Section 1.6, page 8), which are either activities in their own right, or sub-studies associated with a clinical trial or observational study.

A key feature of many laboratory experiments is minimising variability, and this is achieved by careful control of the conditions, including how samples or animals are stored and handled, and how exposures or interventions are administered or delivered. Other important design features are:

- Having replicate measurements on the same sample (also intra-observer variability).
- Repeated measures over time.
- Repeatability, where the same sample is evaluated by different assessors (inter-observer variability).
- Minimising the risk of contaminating samples.
- Minimising or allowing for measurement error.
- Having quality control samples.

These should all be discussed in the study design sections when appropriate.

4.7.1 Study design and conduct

Box 4.11 shows the main areas to cover when describing how a laboratory experiment might be conducted.

Box 4.11 Specific areas of study design to cover when describing laboratory experiments

Section heading	What to cover (when appropriate)
Study subjects	• Types of biological samples (e.g. blood, saliva, urine or tissue), where they will come from, and how they will be stored. • Types of organisms (e.g. bacteria or viruses, and the strain). • For animal experiments, specify the species, sex, strain and age, and the justification for the chosen species, especially if primates are used. • If the samples or animals are to be randomised to an intervention or exposure, details of the allocation method should be specified.
Techniques, interventions or exposures used	• A clear outline of the methodology; the use of standard techniques or whether new ones will be developed as part of the study. • A clear description of what the interventions or exposures are, and how they will be administered, including the dose, frequency and duration. • What reagents or assays will be used? • What equipment will be used? • If free materials or technical equipment are supplied from a commercial company, this should be stated. • Methods for quality control.

Assessments of samples or animals; collecting data	• A detailed description of how the animals or biological samples will be assessed:
	   • What will the measurements be?
	   • What will happen at each time point (such as clinical examinations, biochemical or imaging tests, and any other evaluation)?
	   • The frequency of the assessments.
	   • How long animals will be in the study?

Procedures for handling animals	• How and where will the animals be kept? • The procedures in place to minimise pain and, discomfort. • Procedures for euthanasia.
Safety of researchers	• Describe measures in place to protect laboratory staff from harmful substances or exposures.

4.8 Describing sample size

Specifying the number of subjects, samples or animals for a study is often required, and there is usually a section in the grant application form where the applicants explain or justify this. The sample size can influence the study duration, the level of resources requested and ultimately the financial costs. Sample size estimation is not an exact science. The estimate is only as reliable as the assumptions used, and therefore can only give a rough idea of how big a study should be. It does not matter if one method or set of assumptions yields 500 subjects while another gives 520, because this represents only an extra 10 subjects per trial group. What is important is whether 500 or 700 subjects are needed. For some studies such as clinical trials of children or incapacitated adults, or animal experiments, it is advisable to use the minimum number of subjects that can give a reasonably reliable answer. Sample size is usually based on the primary outcome measure and should be developed in consultation with a statistician.

4.8.1 Assumptions needed for a typical sample size calculation

Qualitative studies tend to be relatively small, and therefore may not need a formal size calculation. Researchers could continue to recruit and interview subjects and collect data until they reach a point of data saturation, that is when the researcher no longer finds any new information. Pilot or feasibility studies (see Section 3.5, page 29) also do not normally require a sample size estimate. For many other types of studies, there are three pieces of information needed to produce the target sample size (Figure 4.3).

- The *effect size* is perhaps the most important parameter (see page 65 for definition), and could come from previous evidence or may be one that is judged to be associated with a minimum clinically important effect. The larger the effect, the smaller the sample size needs to be. However, researchers should not overestimate the magnitude of the effect size, because it is possible that the observed effect at the end of the study will be smaller and therefore not statistically significant, given the smaller sample size. If a surrogate marker (see Section 4.3.1, page 42), is used in a randomised phase II trial, the effect size may need to be larger than that for a corresponding true endpoint. For example, in order to see a hazard ratio for overall survival of about 0.75 in a subsequent cancer trial, a hazard ratio as low as 0.60 might be expected for a surrogate such as progression-free survival.
- The level of *statistical significance* is the chance of finding an effect in the proposed study when in reality one does not exist, so the conclusion of the trial would be wrong; it should be low. Two-sided tests are

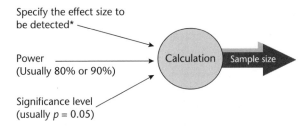

Figure 4.3 Illustration of the information needed to produce a sample size estimate.
* The effect size could be any statistic that is associated with making comparisons (see page 65). for example:
- Two proportions (for the relative risk, odds ratio or risk difference).
  Standardised difference (for the difference between two mean values).
- Two survival rates at a specific time point or two median survival times (for the hazard ratio), plus the length of the recruitment and follow-up periods.
- Correlation or regression coefficient (comparing two continuous measurements).
  Significance level can be smaller than 0.05, such as 0.01 for phase III trials, or larger (e.g. 0.10–0.20) for phase II trials.

always recommended. A one-sided test is appropriate for phase II or non-inferiority clinical trials, or where it is not plausible that an effect can go in either direction (a brief justification should be given in this situation). Applicants should not use one-sided tests just because it gives them a smaller sample size.
- *Power* is the chance of finding an effect size of the magnitude specified (or greater), if it really exists; it should be high.

Box 4.12 shows examples of text that could be used in describing sample size in a grant application. If the study endpoint is a time-to-event measure (e.g. overall survival), the expected number of events should be specified as well as the sample size.

Some researchers specifically choose an effect size to produce what they consider to be a feasible study size. However, they are consequently unable to make firm enough conclusions with the observed results because the sample size is not large enough. In the grant application it is worth justifying the effect size, if possible, with reference to published or unpublished evidence, or by specifying one that is judged to be realistic by most colleagues.

A statistical expert, who will be a member of the funding committee or an external reviewer, will wish to replicate the stated sample size. Applicants should ensure that all the necessary parameters used for the calculation are provided in the application, and it is also worth stating which software was used (if relevant), or give a published reference.

Box 4.12 Examples of wording in sample size sections

Study type	Possible wording*
Case–control study	The study aims to examine the association between maternal smoking and birth defects. About **25%** of women with an unaffected birth are expected to smoke, and we aim to detect an odds ratio of **1.75**. With **80%** power, **5%** **two-sided** test of statistical significance, and that there would be **3** controls per case (i.e. baby with a birth defect), the sample size is 170 cases and 510 controls.
Single-arm phase II clinical trial	The percentage of patients with lung cancer whose tumour shrinks (i.e. complete or partial response) after standard treatment is about **20%**. Drug A should not have a response rate as low as this. It is expected that Drug A would increase the rate to **35%**. A single-arm study would require 44 patients to show an increase from 20% to 35% as statistically significant at the **10%** level (**one-sided**) with **80%** power. If at least 13 patients have a response, this would justify having a larger trial.
Randomised controlled phase II trial	The median survival time using standard treatment is **4** months. New Therapy Q is expected to increase this to **6** months. This is equivalent to a hazard ratio of **0.67**. Assuming the trial has **24** months of recruitment and **12** months follow-up, and there is **80%** power and a **one-sided** test of statistical significance at the **10%** level, 58 patients are required in each group. Total trial size is 116 (which should yield 110 events).
Randomised phase III trial (superiority)	The proportion of elderly individuals who develop flu within 6 months is normally **10%**. It is expected that the flu vaccine would decrease the incidence to **5%**. To detect a difference of 10% versus 5% requires a trial of 580 subjects in each arm (vaccine and placebo), with **90%** power and **two-sided test** of statistical significance at the 5% level. Total trial size is 1160 subjects.
Randomised phase III trial (non-inferiority)	A new pain killer, with fewer side effects, is expected not to be worse than standard treatments. The usual mean pain score on a visual analogue scale (VAS) is **75 mm**, with a standard deviation of **40 mm**. The new drug should not be worse than 85 mm (i.e. the mean VAS needs to be

Study type	Possible wording*
	lower than this), corresponding to a maximum allowable difference of **10 mm**. To show this requires a trial of 340 patients in each arm, with **90**% power and **one-sided test** of statistical significance at the **2.5**% level. Total trial size is 680 patients.
Laboratory experiment	The primary objective is to examine the correlation between Biomarker A and Biomarker B. A moderate correlation coefficient is expected of about **0.35**. To detect this with **80**% power and **two-sided** test of statistical significance at the **5**% level requires 61 samples, each with a value for both biomarkers.

*The numbers (parameters) in bold are the ones used in the calculation to produce the sample size. (The examples given for clinical trials can easily be applied to laboratory experiments.) For the methods and software, see references on page 121 under the section 'Sample size'.

4.8.2 Reasons for increasing the sample size estimate

Once the basic sample size has been calculated (as in Box 4.12), there are times when it is appropriate to increase it, before specifying the actual target in the grant application.

These include:

• Having multiple primary outcome measures, or multiple comparisons, where allowance should be made for increasing the likelihood of finding a chance effect. For example, with three primary endpoints the level of statistical significance used in the sample size estimation could be 0.017 instead of 0.05 (i.e. 0.05/3).

• Allowing for study subjects who drop out of the study (i.e. lost to follow up), meaning that it is not possible to get a value for the main study endpoints (cohort studies and clinical trials).

• Having a factorial controlled clinical trial, used to examine two new interventions, and when an interaction between them is likely.

• Having interim analyses during a clinical trial, i.e. early looks at the main outcome measure.

• Allowing for non-compliance to an intervention in a clinical trial.

• Having failed laboratory samples, in which there is no value for an important measurement.

4.9 Describing the main statistical analyses

Many grant applications will require a summary of the statistical analyses to be performed at the end of the study. Standard analyses will usually apply, for example, observational studies are commonly analysed using multivariate regression techniques that can allow for potential confounders, interactions or effect modifiers. Applicants should ensure that they use the correct one, which depends on the type of outcome measure used: linear, logistic or Cox proportional hazards regressions for continuous, binary/categorical or time-to-event data, respectively. For matched case–control studies, the analysis can allow for the matching factors used in the design. Randomised trials could be analysed using simple methods, such as a comparison of two mean values (*t*-test or Mann–Whitney test), two proportions (chi-squared test) or two survival curves (logrank test); or the multivariate regression methods mentioned above when making adjustments for other factors. When repeated measures are used in the study (i.e. the same endpoint is measured on several different occasions from the same study subject or specimen), an appropriate method of analysis should be specified such as repeated measures analysis of variance or mixed modelling. If non-standard statistical analyses are proposed, they should be described in some detail.

The name of a statistician should be provided in the grant application; as a member of the Study Team, as a collaborator, or someone who has given advice on the methods and sample size before submission. A funding body may want reassurance that the study has been developed with sufficient statistical expertise, so it is worth asking someone with experience to help write or comment on relevant sections of the grant application, particularly on sample size and statistical analysis.

The analysis associated with each primary objective and primary endpoint needs to be clearly specified, and it should be consistent with the method of sample size calculation. For example, in the example of the flu vaccine in Boxes 4.9 and 4.12, the primary endpoint is the proportion of people who develop clinician-diagnosed influenza within 6 months, so the main analysis would be a comparison of two proportions (i.e. relative risk or risk difference); an analysis based on *the time until* the person developed flu, which produces a hazard ratio, would be inconsistent with the sample size method. Sometimes it is helpful to list the statistical analytical methods for each objective and its corresponding outcome measure(s) in turn.

In observational studies, it may be necessary to discuss briefly how potential confounding factors or biases would be examined. For laboratory experiments, when there are many comparisons or factors to consider, it might be worth describing methods for allowing for this, such as Bonferroni corrections. In clinical trials of new interventions, there are three key items to cover in the analysis: efficacy, safety and treatment compliance. There may also be analyses associated with health-related quality of life or health economic analyses, and these too should be described briefly.

Most research studies produce an *effect size*; a single quantitative summary measure obtained by comparing an endpoint between two groups, or by comparing two different measurements on the same group of subjects/ samples. They allow the results to be interpreted and communicated more easily. Examples are relative risk, odds ratio, hazard ratio, absolute risk difference, difference between two mean or median values, and regression or correlation coefficients.

4.9.1 An example

Each outcome measure should be associated with an objective, and all endpoints should be clearly defined. The following could be associated with a randomised trial comparing two interventions (the method of analysis for each endpoint is stated briefly):

Endpoints
Overall survival: taken from the date of randomisation until the date of death from any cause; those who have not died will be censored at the date they were last seen alive.

Treatment compliance: patients who complete the full course of the trial treatments, as specified in the protocol.

Analysis
Overall survival will be analysed using Kaplan–Meier curves and the logrank test, and hazard ratios estimated with 95% confidence intervals and p-values. The hazard ratio will also be adjusted for other factors (i.e. age and gender used to stratify subjects in the randomisation) using Cox proportional hazards regression.

The proportion of patients who complete treatment will be compared between the two trial groups using a chi-squared test. Reasons for not completing treatment will also be summarised for each group.

4.9.2 Interim or futility analysis for phase III clinical trials

Some trials have interim analyses for superiority built into the design, often with stopping guidelines based on p-values. This involves discontinuing recruitment early because there is already a clear and statistically significant treatment difference. It should be specified when these analyses are scheduled to occur (e.g. after half the patients have been recruited and followed up for 6 months, or half the number of events have been observed), and what size of p-value is required to justify early termination (many trials use a cut-off of <0.001).

Furthermore, not all phase III studies produce a positive result, so it might be worth having a *futility analysis*. This is also an early analysis of the data conducted when, for example, the first third or half of trial subjects have been recruited and had a reasonable length of follow-up (there could be another one or two futility analyses later in the trial). The observed results can indicate whether the new intervention is highly likely to be either ineffective or the effect is much weaker than originally anticipated (and so may not be clinically worthwhile). Statistical methods exist that can use the data collected so far to estimate the probability of finding a specified clinically meaningful effect if the trial continued to the end (e.g. Whitehead & Matsushita 2003). If this probability is very low, for example <10%, then it might not be worth continuing. Such analyses could be particularly useful if the proposed trial is quite large (e.g. >1000 subjects), when the prior evidence on efficacy is not very strong, or the disorder of interest is uncommon.

The decision to stop early is usually made by an Independent Data Monitoring Committee (IDMC, see Section 2.5, page 21) who have all the necessary data to examine, such as any clinical benefit observed so far, and safety and accrual, including unblinded data for double-blind trials.

An advantage of an interim or futility analysis is that it can lead to the study being stopped early. This avoids recruiting more subjects to a trial in which a clear treatment effect is already found, or one that is likely to be negative (which has ethical implications because those allocated to the new intervention are unlikely to benefit). The researchers can thus save time and resources, and instead concentrate on developing different studies. Ultimately there is a significant cost saving to the funding body. However, one of the main limitations of futility analyses is that current data is used to forecast what *might* happen if the study continued, and it is probably not appropriate for relatively small studies (say <200 subjects) or where the accrual rate is so high that by the time the early patients have been followed up and the futility analysis performed, the cumulative recruitment is not far from the full target. Also, reliably examining treatment effects in important subgroups, as part of an interim or futility analysis, is difficult because there may not be a reasonable number of recruited subjects. Grant applicants should therefore consider whether specifying an early analysis as part of the study design might strengthen the application. Box 4.13 is an example of the wording that could be used for a futility analysis.

> **Box 4.13** Example of text used to describe futility in a phase III clinical trial for an uncommon disorder
>
> *Sample size and futility analysis*:
> The expected median overall survival in patients given the control treatment is approximately 12 months. The new treatment is expected to increase this to 17 months, that is a hazard ratio of 0.70. Assuming a recruitment period of 5 years and 18 months of follow-up after the end of recruitment, we require 300 patients (259 events), with 80% power and 5% level of statistical significance. This disorder is uncommon, so we realistically expect to randomise about five patients per month.
> A futility analysis will be performed after half of the patients have been recruited ($n = 150$) and followed up for 6 months. This will be used to determine whether the new treatment is highly unlikely to be effective. Accrual to the trial will continue during the 6-month follow-up, when only a further 30 patients would be recruited. Futility guidelines will be developed in partnership with the IDMC. Statistical methods for futility will be applied to the observed data to estimate the probability of finding a hazard ratio of 0.70 or lower if the trial continued to the end. A low probability of less than 10% would be used in support of stopping early. Other factors may also be considered by the IDMC, such as adverse events and accrual rates.

4.9.3 Monitoring safety in clinical trials

The Study Team, and staff who recruit and manage subjects at participating centres, should always monitor safety during the trial, when appropriate. There is usually very close monitoring of subjects who are in early phase I and II trials of investigational drugs. Also, one of the key functions of an IDMC (see page 21) is to examine adverse events, and recommend a trial stops early if there is unacceptable harm. Safety monitoring is useful for interventions such as investigational drugs, exposures such as radiotherapy, and surgical techniques. Other interventions, for example, those associated with a change in behaviour or lifestyle factors are often not expected to cause adverse events.

Applicants sometimes provide a *stopping rule* for safety in clinical trials. This is usually a single numerical cut-off, i.e. if a pre-specified number of subjects in a particular intervention group suffer a serious adverse event then the study should be terminated early. The words 'stopping rule' imply something that is inflexible, so that once the single pre-specified criterion is met, the trial must be terminated. However, 'stopping guidelines' may be a more

appropriate phrase, because early termination is an important decision that should depend on several factors, including:
- The proportion of subjects affected with an adverse event, and whether this could be due to chance.
- The specific types of events seen, their severity and how easily they are treated.
- The type of subjects/patients in the trial (e.g. fit and healthy, or generally unfit or elderly).
- Any clinical benefit seen.

In phase I healthy volunteer trials, it is usually quite easy to identify adverse events caused by the trial treatment. However, in early phase trials of people who are already ill, for example with cancer, the research team needs to distinguish serious adverse events that are caused by the trial treatment and those associated with the disease itself or any concomitant therapies.

Applicants should consider whether it is appropriate to specify a process for safety monitoring, especially for early phase trials of unlicensed therapies or those with expected serious side effects. Dose-escalation phase I studies already have safety monitoring built in. For randomised phase III trials with a control group, it is possible to compare adverse event rates with the new intervention during the trial, and if a difference emerges that is statistically significant, consideration could be given to whether it is appropriate to stop the study (or just stop one of the groups in trials with several new interventions). For single-arm or randomised controlled phase II trials, a stopping guideline for the group could be provided (see below).

Safety monitoring often involves pre-specifying in the application what would be an unacceptable percentage of subjects who suffer a (serious) side effect, and in some cases it might be appropriate to list the side effects of interest.[6] The following text is one way of describing safety monitoring for an early phase clinical trial. It is based on a randomised phase II trial for a cancer (comparing a new treatment with standard therapy), with a target sample size of 56 patients per group, but part of it could also be used for a single-arm trial:

> *A treatment-related grade 3 or 4 toxicity rate of more than 30% would be considered unacceptable in the new treatment group (using the National Cancer Institute Common Terminology Criteria for Adverse Events, an internationally recognised grading system). As soon as*

---

[6] Because people who are already ill may develop certain adverse events anyway, so interest is in unexpected events, or perhaps the worsening of those that are expected.

17 patients in this group suffer a grade 3 or 4 event (this is 30% of n = 56), this would trigger us to review the safety data more regularly with the IDMC. If at least 24 patients have a grade 3 or 4 event, this would be used to help decide whether the trial stops early, because the likelihood of this occurring by chance, if the underlying rate really is 30%, is small (p = 0.03). Observing 24 patients would indicate that the true rate is probably greater than 30%. Because the trial is randomised, we will also compare the toxicity rates between the arms, to confirm whether the rate is indeed higher in one arm than the other. There will be a regular IDMC review of safety data (at least once per year, or more frequently if required).

4.10 Systematic reviews

The previous sections were associated with individual studies. However, some funding organisations will provide a grant to conduct a systematic review of the accumulation of evidence in a particular area, in order to provide a clearer view on the effectiveness of a particular intervention, or risk or causal factor (Glasziou et al. 2001, Khan et al. 2003). The outcome measure from each study is quantitatively combined using a statistical technique called *meta-analysis*. Such reviews, which are commonly performed for studies of humans, are based on identifying published and unpublished studies on the same subject. They could be used for one of the following purposes:

- To confirm existing practice but provide a more precise estimate of a treatment effect or risk factor. Also, subgroup analyses are based on more subjects than in any individual study, and so have greater statistical power, though spurious effects could still be found by chance if many subgroups are examined.
- To change existing practice. Occasionally, systematic reviews have led to a new intervention being adopted into practice, but usually they have resulted in an existing treatment becoming more commonly used. Reviews based on observational studies usually help to identify new risk factors for a disorder or early death. Systematic reviews can be used to develop guidelines for defining standard clinical practice or developing public health education policies.

By design, the effects of bias and confounding should be minimised in clinical trials, especially in double-blind trials. However, applicants should be aware that an observational study could be affected by bias and confounding, and so a meta-analysis of several studies with the same biases and confounders could just magnify the effects of these two factors and produce a spurious association that appears to be precise (narrow confidence interval). Therefore, in the grant application it would be worth describing how potential bias and confounding might be dealt with.

There are two types of systematic reviews: those in which all the information is extracted from published or unpublished articles (i.e. the meta-analysis is based on summary results) and those where the lead researcher of each constituent study is contacted, the raw data requested and the systematic reviewers perform a full statistical analysis. The latter is called an *individual patient data (IPD)* meta-analysis, and this type tends to be more likely to be funded. Box 4.14 shows the main areas to cover when considering a systematic review.

Box 4.14 Specific areas to cover when describing systematic reviews

Section heading	What to cover (when appropriate)

Eligibility of studies	• Specify how potential studies would be identified:
	  • Which electronic databases would be searched, for example MEDLINE, EMBASE, PUBMED
	  • The keywords to be used.
	• The grant applicants should conduct a preliminary literature search, and describe what was found, including an estimate of the number of studies that might be included in the final analysis.

Extraction of data	• Specify the outcome measures and any other variables to be obtained from each study (i.e. from the published report, or from the original research group who conducted the study when using an IPD meta-analysis). • Specify how allowance might be made for potential confounders or biases (observational studies).

Analysis	• Specify the methods of statistical analysis (meta-analysis):
	  • Investigation of heterogeneity
	  • Perhaps mention that both fixed and random effects models would be examined
	  • Indicate whether any subgroup analyses would be performed.
	• Describe non-standard analyses (eg dose-response modelling, or combining data from randomised trials with observational studies)

Summary points

- Try to avoid overly technical language, jargon and abbreviations.
- Clearly specify the study objectives (hypotheses) and define the corresponding outcome measures (study endpoints), and try not to confuse the two.
- Each objective should be described using one succinct sentence.
- Clearly specify the type of study design to be used, and justify the choice where appropriate.
- Ensure that all the key design features or methodological attributes of the study are described.
- Design the study with realistic objectives in mind, and ensure that the study, as designed, can meet these.
- For clinical trials of interventions, especially those with expected adverse side effects, specify a process for monitoring and dealing with serious adverse events.
- Consider carefully the study size and duration.
- Produce a concise abstract that is easy to read and understand.

Chapter 5 **Associated documents with the grant application**

The main sections required in a typical grant application form were presented in Chapters 3 and 4. Some funding organisations also request other documentation to be included with the application form, and this will be specified in the information on the website or as a checklist to complete. Applicants should ensure that all such requested documents are sent by the deadline. Failure to omit one could mean that consideration of the application is deferred to the next funding committee meeting, which may be several months later. If any of the documents might not be ready in time, the applicants should check with the funding body whether it is acceptable to send them after the deadline. Sometimes the administrative staff at the funding body will inform the applicants if there is anything missing from a submission and hopefully allow it to be forwarded [See also 'Covering letter', page 100].

5.1 Study protocol

Most studies require a protocol before they can start. This is a document intended for use by the Study Team and all the centres participating in the study. It describes some or all of the following (when appropriate):
- The background to and justification for the study.
- The objectives and outcome measures.
- The study design, including methods, sample size, and statistical analysis.
- How subjects are to be recruited, managed and treated.
- How biological samples or imaging scans are to be collected, stored and analysed.
- Procedures for monitoring the safety and well-being of humans and animals.
- Procedures for protecting research staff from hazardous substances in laboratory experiments.
- The technical and laboratory methods to be used.

How to Write a Grant Application, 1st edition. © Allan Hackshaw. Published 2011 by Blackwell Publishing Ltd.

The protocol is essential when applying for approval to conduct studies of humans and animals, for example, to research and ethics committees (in Europe), and Institutional Review Boards (in the US and Japan). Protocols are also necessary for clinical trials of humans, because additional approvals are required from the national regulatory agencies (for example, a Competent Authority from each country in Europe; and the Food and Drug Administration in the US).

Not all funding organisations require a study protocol, because the application form should already contain the necessary information needed to evaluate the proposal. However, the protocol is sometimes used instead of a comprehensive and structured form (eg. for commercial companies). The format depends on the type of study proposed, but will include items already discussed in Chapter 3, namely the background and justification, and those given in Boxes 4.6, 4.11 and 4.12 (in Chapter 4). Applicants should also be aware of any national regulations or special procedures that may apply to the study, such as for animal experiments, clinical trials on humans, or studies on children or incapacitated adults, and perhaps indicate this in the study protocol.

If a protocol is submitted as part of a funding application it does not have to be the final version, because suggested changes made by the funding committee may need to be incorporated. Even after a project proposal is funded, subsequent changes could still be made after comments from the Institutional Review Board, or research or ethics committees. However, the protocol should be clear and well written.

After a project is funded, there are occasionally major changes during the study to the objectives, design or interventions. For example, one of the interventions in a clinical trial may be changed, or the target sample size is significantly increased or decreased. The applicants are usually obliged to inform the funding organisation of this, and the protocol changed accordingly (see also Section 8.1, page 115).

5.2 Participant Information Sheet

For studies on humans, a Participant Information Sheet[1] (PIS) is given to potential subjects, or their legal representative, who must give informed consent before taking part. This is a legal requirement in many countries, particularly for clinical trials of investigational drugs. Sufficient information must be provided about the study to allow subjects to examine what will happen to them, and to assess the possible benefits and risks of taking part. Suggested sections are shown in Box 5.1.

---

[1] The term 'Patient Information Sheet' is normally used when the subjects are already ill.

Box 5.1 Suggested sections in a Participant Information Sheet

- Background and justification for the study.
- A description of how subjects will be selected (or if a clinical trial, how they would be randomised, and the probability of being in each treatment arm).
- A description of the trial interventions, especially identifying those that are experimental and unlicensed for use in humans (clinical trials only).
- What the subject has to do as part of the study and the expected duration of their participation (including what the assessments are, and how frequent).
- Which biological samples (eg. blood, saliva, urine, or tissue), if any, are being collected, and what will be done with them for the purpose of the trial and for future research.
- What are the possible side effects of the interventions, including the magnitude of the risks, and discomforts to the subject, as well as to any embryo, fetus or nursing infant of the subject (clinical trials only).
- The possible benefits and disadvantages of taking part.
- Alternative procedures or treatments available to the subject if they do not participate.
- A statement about securing confidentiality of data, and who will have access to the data and for how long; also what personal data (eg full names or contact addresses) will be used and by whom.
- A statement that participation is voluntary and refusal to participate will involve no penalty or loss of benefit; and that the subject may withdraw at any time.
- Circumstances under which a subject's participation may be terminated by the investigator without regard to the subject's consent.
- Who is funding the research?
- Who to contact during the study if there are any queries.
- A statement about liability and compensation if a subject is harmed by being in the study.

The PIS must be written as clearly as possible, because participants will come from the general population and most are unlikely to have specialist knowledge. Subjects may decline to take part if the text is confusing. Additionally, there may be centre or country-specific requirements, such as insurance and indemnity. Writing a good PIS can be difficult, so it is advisable to ask several people to comment on the text, particularly for complex studies, such as clinical trials with several arms. A draft could also be given to someone who would be eligible for the study (such as a former patient), or a representative of a relevant patient or consumer group. A research nurse, who already has experience of dealing with subjects who are similar to those proposed for the study, is in an ideal position to comment because they are often the ones involved in recruitment.

A draft version of the PIS is often requested by the funding body, but may change in response to comments from the funding committee or at a later stage (ie. the institutional, research or ethics committees). The PIS is required to have several sections, and depending on the complexity of the proposed study could cover five to ten pages.

It is a useful document because it describes the study objectives and design in a clear way, with minimal technical terms that would otherwise appear in the application form or study protocol. Funding committee members therefore often use the PIS to understand the proposal, and non-scientific members of the committee find it especially helpful. Sometimes parts of the application form are much easier to understand in the PIS. Applicants need to ensure that the sections on study objectives, design and conduct in the application form (or protocol) are consistent with the text in the PIS.

5.3 Curricula vitae of the Chief Investigator and all co-applicants

The funding body usually requires up-to-date curricula vitae for the named Chief Investigator and co-applicants (co-investigators). A full curriculum vitae (CV) for each individual is not needed, and the application form will either have a pre-formatted CV section or will specify what to include. The required items are generally:

- Qualifications (degree level and above).
- Current and previous employment – positions held, academic titles (if relevant), and names of employers.
- Area of expertise, for example clinician, statistician, scientist, psychologist, or health economist.
- The number of published peer-reviewed articles.
- Selected references – not all published references over the whole career are required; it may be sufficient to include only those in the past five years that are relevant to the application.
- Grant applications already held, either as Chief or co-investigator – only summary items are needed (ie. project title, names of the investigators, total amount of funding, funding body, and study period).

5.4 Letters of support from co-applicants, centre investigators, collaborators, or other advisors

Many studies are conducted at multiple sites (ie multicentre) and will therefore require input from several professionals or experts on a specific aspect of the project (see Sections 2.1 and 2.2, pages 15 and 19). There may be one or more sections in the grant application where the names of all the co-applicants, centre investigators and collaborators could be listed. Funding bodies also tend to require a copy of a signed letter of support from each investigator or collaborator to the Chief Investigator to be enclosed with the grant application. The letter need only be a single page, with two or three sentences stating that the collaborator has seen the study proposal and is willing to participate. The letter does not formally obligate the collaborator to take part in the study, but when the project involves recruiting human subjects, it can significantly help the funding committee to evaluate the feasibility of recruitment (see Section 3.5). If a large cohort study or clinical trial has a target sample size of, for example, 500 subjects but few or no collaborators listed on the application, the funding body may query the likelihood of this target being met.

5.5 Letters of support from commercial companies

Some studies, usually clinical trials of investigational drugs or products, and laboratory experiments, require products or materials from a commercial company. This could be a free drug or medical device, or key materials or technical equipment essential for the study. Occasionally, the commercial company will also provide some funds to help with study co-ordination, or costs at recruiting centres, such as additional clinical visits and assessments incurred as a result of the study. In these cases, the applicant must enclose a letter of support from the company with the grant application. The letter does not usually have to be long and detailed, and although it may not be a legally binding formal commitment to the study, it needs to indicate a firm willingness to provide the drug or materials for free. The funding committee will want to see evidence of this because without these products the study cannot go ahead. Applicants should allow sufficient time before the application deadline for initial discussion with the company, and for the company representatives to review the proposal and draft the letter of support. Occasionally, the funding committee approval is conditional on a formal commitment by the company, and no funds will be released to the applicants before this is provided. If the grant application is successful, the researchers will then enter further negotiations with the company over the details of the study[2] and agreement, before the company signs a contract, which is usually legally binding.

5.6 Other documents specific to the field of research

The funding body guidelines will specify clearly what other documents are required, and this list must be examined and adhered to carefully. Studies associated with, for example, animal experiments, gene therapy, recombinant DNA, or those that involve hazardous chemicals or exposures, may require a copy of any appropriate regulatory licences or certificates held by the research unit in which the proposed study will be conducted. If a certain document may take longer than expected to obtain, the applicant should inform the administrative staff at the funding body, who may allow some flexibility on its submission. Such documents are not usually needed by the external reviewers or funding committee for their evaluation, but rather the funding organisation needs to check that the planned study can indeed go ahead.

Summary points

- Check with the funding body, or information from their website or other documentation, which associated documents need to be submitted with the grant application form.
- For studies of humans, try to submit a draft version of the Participant Information Sheet. Ask a research nurse, patient or consumer representative to review the draft before submission.
- Ensure that curricula vitae of all the co-applicants are up-to-date and included in the application.
- Allow sufficient time to obtain letters of support from key collaborators (who are not co-applicants), centre investigators, or commercial companies who are providing free materials or equipment.

---

[2] The company will have an internal review of the study protocol to ensure it is consistent with their own policies or procedures associated with the product.

Chapter 6 **Financial costs**

Once the justification, objectives and design have been considered and drafted, the applicants should be in a good position to contemplate the financial costs to request from the funding organisation. It can be difficult to formulate an accurate estimate of costs, especially for individuals who are relatively new to research. It is important not to underestimate the costs, particularly those associated with setting up a study, which can take several months.

If an application is successful, the whole grant is not usually paid to the host institution at the start of the study. The host institution will invoice the funding body each year. The claimed costs should be similar to those specified in the financial section of the grant application form, but if they are noticeably higher, the funding body will need to review and approve them, often after discussion with the Study Team or administrative staff at the host institution.

6.1 Overview of items to include in the financial costs

There are three main categories of costs, and most projects require funds to cover each of these:
1 Staff.
2 Running or recurring expenses (non-staff costs that need to be met each year during the study), for example, printing and consumables or laboratory materials.
3 One-off costs for materials, equipment or services.

Table 6.1 shows examples of items typically requested on a grant application, according to the type of study. These are all referred to as *direct costs*, because they apply to staff, items or activities used specifically for the proposed study. There are also *indirect costs* or *overheads* which may be added to the grant

How to Write a Grant Application, 1st edition. © Allan Hackshaw. Published 2011 by Blackwell Publishing Ltd.

Table 6.1 Examples of commonly requested items on a grant application, according to type of study*

Category of costs	Observational study	Clinical trial on humans	Laboratory experiment
Staff	• Study co-ordinator. • Epidemiologist. • Research fellow, assistant or nurse. • Qualitative researcher. • Statistician. • Data manager. • Administrative/clerical staff. • IT and database support.	• Study co-ordinator. • Research assistant/nurse. • Statistician. • Pathologist. • Data manager/monitor. • Administrative/clerical staff. • Health economist. • Training or clinical fellows. • IT and database support.	• Research technician. • Laboratory technician. • Postdoctoral research fellows or assistants. • Clinical research fellows.
Running or recurring expenses (that occur for more than 1 year of the study)	• Office expenses, e.g. stationery postage, and printing. • Travel and subsistence for meetings with the study team and collaborators. • Any clinical assessments, imaging scans, or other measurements.	• Office expenses, e.g. stationery postage, and printing. • Travel and subsistence for meetings with the study team, collaborators and oversight committees. • Collection, storage and analysis of biological samples or imaging scans.	• Laboratory materials, e.g. syringes, assays, reagents, microarrays. • Obtaining and maintaining animals. • Storage and analysis of biological samples. • Annual cost of maintenance and repair of laboratory equipment.

(Continued)

Table 6.1 (Continued)

Category of costs	Observational study	Clinical trial on humans	Laboratory experiment
	• Collection, storage and analysis of biological samples. • Central pathology or imaging reviews.	• Any extra clinical assessments, scans or other measurements. • Renewing national regulatory approvals. • Labelling, packaging and distribution of investigational drugs. • Central pathology or imaging reviews.	• Office expenses, e.g. stationery, postage, and printing. • Travel and subsistence for meetings with the study team and collaborators. • Staff training. • Systems to protect staff from hazardous chemicals or exposures.
Fixed one-off costs	• Health economics. • Statistical support. • Computers and software licenses. • Retrieving data from regional or national databases, or patient records. • Freezers for storing samples.	• Health economics. • Statistical support. • National regulatory approvals (trials of investigational drugs). • Computers and licenses. • Retrieving data from regional or national databases. • Pharmacy set-up fees (drug trials). • Freezers for storing samples.	• Laboratory equipment. • Freezers for storing samples. • Computers and licenses. • Consultancies from specialists.

*Some items can be listed as either staff or fixed one-off costs. Choosing which is more appropriate depends on the size of the study and the expected amount of input that may be required (see Section 6.4); eg statistical support could be requested as staff for large studies, or one-off costs for small studies. A funding body may not provide costs for some items listed.

application (see Section 6.2). All costs should be properly justified in the application. Running expenses for printing, postage and stationery can be combined without further breakdown, unless the total per year seems excessive. With increasing reliance on email and electronic documents accessed via the Internet, printing costs may not need to be as high as they were several years ago.

Many host institutions will have their own financial algorithm that produces an estimate of costs for each year of the study, which allows for any year-on-year increases, such as inflation or staff pay rises.[1] Some institutions have internal software that can be used. The Study Team should, where possible, ensure that they have used this algorithm when specifying the breakdown of costs requested in the grant application.

The amount of money requested for each staff member or study activity will often depend on several general considerations, as well as what the funding body is prepared to cover:

- The study size and duration.
- How much data is to be collected, and whether this will be entered onto a database by hand, or will be transferred electronically.
- The complexity of the study or laboratory experiment, and whether large and expensive equipment is required.
- Consumables, such as printing, or laboratory materials.
- Costs of drug manufacturing, labelling and distribution.
- Costs of collecting and storing biological samples, as part of the main study or as a translational research sub-study; and costs for laboratory analyses or central review of imaging scans or pathology reports (see Section 4.3.2, page 43).
- Travel for members of the Study Team, staff named on the grant, or for collaborators to meet the Study Team.
- Professional development (i.e. training) and attending conferences for staff on the grant.

For large studies, such as cohort studies or clinical trials of humans, a crude approach is to divide the total cost requested by the target number of subjects; ie. a cost per subject (or per patient) recruited. If this seems very high, applicants should either try to reduce the costs or clearly justify in the application why all are essential to the study. Furthermore, when collecting biological samples for analysis several years later, there might need to be a cost for long-term storage, for example, freezers, and their maintenance and replacement. Sometimes, the total cost (overall or per year) is clearly too high, so the applicants must prioritise which items are essential for the study, and remove others.

---

[1] Not all funding bodies will accept inflationary or salary increments.

Many funding bodies have a maximum monetary limit per study per year, and this would be stated in their documentation. If the costs for a proposed study exceed this slightly, it might be acceptable for good applications to proceed, but if the costs are significantly greater, the applicants should discuss this with senior administrative staff at the funding organisation *before* submitting their application.

Researchers should avoid having excessive direct costs, or requesting money that would be used for projects other than that proposed. The funding organisation and committee members will generally have a good idea of what the expected costs are likely to be for a particular study.

Applicants may believe that if the proposed costs are low their project is likely to be successful, but this could mean that they will not have enough funds to finish the study, and will therefore have to apply later for a grant extension (see Chapter 8). If the application for the extension fails, the researchers will have to find funds elsewhere in order to finish. However, if the initial proposed costs are too high, the funding committee may consider this unfavourably, and applications have failed because of overly inflated costs.

6.2 Indirect costs or overheads (full economic costs)

Most academic institutions, that would eventually host the study if successfully funded, require *overheads* or *indirect costs* to be included in the grant application. The combined direct and indirect costs can be referred to as *full economic costs (FECs)*. The basic principle of FEC is that the true cost of conducting a study to the host institution is greater than that claimed for staff costs or running expenses specifically for the study. To avoid having a significant financial deficit, the host institution needs to recoup as much of the full costs as possible from the funding body, in order to maintain its research portfolio. Overheads would be used to help cover infrastructure, including rent of office or laboratory space, electricity, heating and lighting, and maintenance of central resources such as library services, general estates and facilities, and human resources and finance. Indirect costs may also include the cost of the time spent on the project by the Chief Investigator or other co-applicants based within the host institution, even if they are already receiving a full salary.

Some funding organisations (e.g. charities) do not pay indirect costs at all, others only pay a fixed percentage of the direct costs (40% or 80%), and the rest will pay whatever the host institution estimates the indirect costs to be.

Overheads are based on the direct costs (usually staff). If overheads are calculated as a fixed percentage of the direct costs, for example 40%, a study requiring £200,000 to pay for staff would be associated with £80,000 indirect costs.

The applicants specify a FEC of £280,000 on the grant application (but there should always be a breakdown of direct and indirect costs). The extra £80,000 does not usually go to the research unit conducting the study, but rather to the central finance department at the host institution.[2] When host institutions use a financial algorithm to estimate indirect costs it can also incorporate input from co-applicants and how much laboratory or office space is expected to be used (see Sections 6.8.1 and 6.9.2 for examples). The algorithm could vary between different host institutions. Costs can be calculated by the finance department, but even when this is not the case, it is always checked by them, so it is important that the applicants allow sufficient time for this to be done before the application has to be submitted to the funding body. Once the indirect costs are estimated, the host institution will claim some or all of it from the funding body (in addition to the direct costs), depending on the type of funder; for example, 100% from a commercially funded study or 80% if it is government-funded.

An issue may arise when a commercial company or private benefactor is only willing to pay a certain amount for an academic-sponsored study, and adding overheads far exceeds this. The applicants should discuss the matter with the company or benefactor, and with the finance department of the host institution, to see if a compromise can be reached.

Applicants should also check whether all types of staff requested on a grant are eligible for indirect costs from a particular funding body, because the host institution will want to maximise the amount of overheads it receives. For example, in some cases indirect costs may only apply to research posts, not clerical or administrative posts. The funding committee and external reviewers tend to focus on the direct costs in a grant application. If successful, it will then be up to the funding body to determine how the indirect costs are dealt with.

6.3 Per patient (or per subject) payments

Occasionally, some centres (sites) which recruit individuals to clinical trials or cohort studies may request or be awarded a *per patient* (or *per subject*) *payment*. This is common when a commercial company sponsors and conducts a clinical trial. The payment to the centre is intended to cover:

- The administrative work arising from the study (e.g. study set-up and conduct).
- The time spent by local staff on recruiting and managing patients.

---

[2]Occasionally, the research unit may be given some of this if all the central costs of the host institution are met.

- Any extra assessments or evaluations of the subjects that would not normally be done as part of standard practice (e.g. extra clinic visits, imaging scans or blood tests).
- The costs of other (licensed and standard) therapies that may need to be given at the same time as the new intervention.

Such payments can help greatly to encourage centres to participate, and may therefore boost recruitment. For clinical trials, this could be as much as £2000 or more per patient or subject, depending on the administrative workload required at each centre and the extra assessments for each patient. For studies that are academic-led and academic-sponsored, but funded by a commercial company, the investigators should discuss with the company representatives whether a per patient payment is possible, in addition to free drug or medical devices and the costs of trial co-ordination and data management. Even a nominal amount (e.g. £200–500) would be useful to participating centres. Sometimes, a commercial company pays a single per patient fee, which is intended to cover all the costs (study co-ordination and payments to centres), so the Study Team must decide how such payments are allocated to each participating centre, and how much it keeps within the host institution.

Although many funding organisations, such as charities, do not normally provide per patient or subject costs, applicants should check this with administrative staff at the funding body, because a small payment to centres is always worthwhile.

6.4 Staff costs

Salaries usually represent the highest proportion of the total cost of a study, especially for large studies. Applicants need to specify the grade and cost of each staff member, and how much time they will spend on the project. This is sometimes given as *full-time equivalents (FTEs)* or *whole-time equivalents (WTEs)*. A person who will work every day on the project for the whole study period would be classified as 1.0 FTE. Someone who would work part time, for example, 1 day per week, would be 0.2 FTE; and 2.5 days per week 0.5 FTE. Part-time staff could work regularly for part of the week each week during the whole year, or they could be full time for only part of the year. For example, a health economist may be specified as 0.5 FTE in the final year of the study, but may work full time for 6 months.

When several full-time staff are requested on a grant application, the researchers should ensure that there really will be enough work for each person during each year of the study.

The grade of each post would normally be influenced by guidelines within the host institution, ie. there is likely to be fixed grades for specific types of posts. Applicants should also allow for yearly increases in salary, taking into consideration inflation or mandatory pay rises if staff are on a salary scale which automatically increases each year (usually until a maximum is reached). Normally, it is only necessary to specify the salary range (or band) for each post requested in the application, but a single salary grade (or point) is needed to estimate costs for the study. This can be done using the middle of the salary range for each staff member requested on the grant. If an application is successful, funding organisations, such as governmental bodies, research foundations and charities, usually pay for whoever is actually employed. The salary could be lower or higher than that used in the grant application, depending on the experience of the appointed candidate, but it must be within the salary band specified in the application. In each year of the study, the host institution will invoice the funding body for a certain amount to cover the costs and any approved salary increases.

When researchers seek a grant from a commercial company, they could use the upper limit of the salary band of each post requested, because the company may want to know the maximum costs of the study upfront. If, for example, a salary of £30,000 were used in the application, it might be difficult to invoice the company for £40,000 if a more experienced candidate were appointed.

The extent of some funding support, such as for a statistician, health economist or pathologist, will depend on how much input is required from that post. For large studies, these roles might be involved throughout the study and have had significant input into the design and conduct. Such support may therefore be requested under staff costs; for example, a statistician to analyse interim data and prepare annual reports for an IDMC, see page 21. In smaller studies, this kind of support may be provided as a consultancy, or may be limited to the end of the study when the analyses would be performed. In such cases, these positions may only be required for a few months, and it might be more appropriate to provide a fixed figure under one-off costs, rather than claiming for a staff member under staff costs.

When specifying the staff costs, applicants also need to be aware of any additional costs associated with the actual posts. The salary for a certain position within a salary range is what would be paid directly to the person in post. However, there may be other costs, such as health, national insurance or pension contributions, which must be added to this salary. These are sometimes called *salary on-costs*. They may be 25% of the salary, but the financial algorithm will calculate this exactly. For example, if the salary to be paid to a person is £30,000 in 1 year, and on-costs are £7,500 (these do not go to the staff member, but to the employer or host institution), the total cost requested from the funding body would be £37,500. On-costs may also allow for maternity or sick leave.

The Chief Investigator and co-investigators are not normally expected to include a financial cost for their time spent on the project in the application because they are usually already in full-time paid occupation. However, if a co-investigator will need assistance in their work for the project, costings for a junior staff member may be included. For example, if an experienced statistician is one of the co-investigators, there could still be an item for statistical support in the grant application to pay for a junior statistician to be overseen by the senior statistician. The funding body, or type of grant, will specify whether or not applicants can claim costs for their time in the application. Sometimes, at least one of the applicants is funded entirely or partly on the grant application, often for a programme grant or a large project grant, because they will spend a significant amount of time on the study. This type of cost is included in the indirect costs to the host institution when they cannot be claimed as direct costs from the funding body.

6.4.1 Remote data entry (web-based data entry systems)

Traditionally, many multicentre observational studies and clinical trials relied on paper case report forms (CRFs, see Section 6.8) to be completed by hand at the recruiting centre and then sent to the co-ordinating centre, where the data are entered manually onto a central database. However, studies are increasingly able to use *remote data entry* software systems (electronic CRFs). Staff in recruiting centres log on to the central database and enter data directly, avoiding the use of paper CRFs and central manual data entry in the co-ordinating centre. Many pharmaceutical companies use this approach for their clinical trials. If remote data entry is to be used, the central data management support requested on the grant application should be reduced in comparison with a study using paper CRFs. However, this might need to be partly compensated for by an increased level of IT expertise required to maintain the database system and its security, and possibly the system development costs at the start of the study (if not already in place), including the purchasing of dedicated servers and software.

6.5 Access to core funds and resources

A common problem faced by many researchers is a lack of access to core resources, which can reduce the amount they request on the grant application. Many academic groups, such as a clinical trials unit or disease-specific research unit, have central support, which includes core staff and running expenses. They are often funded from a governmental or charitable organisation, through a programme grant which is reviewed and renewed, for example, every 5 years. These resources are in place regardless of how many studies are being conducted, and can include clinical research fellows, a range of academic staff and research assistants, laboratory scientists, statisticians, IT and database staff, study co-ordinators, data managers and clerical staff. The value of having core resources is that it can help minimise the amount of funding requested for a specific project grant. Large studies, such as cohort studies or clinical trials, often take several months to set up, and some researchers can use core resources for study set-up activities, some follow-up, and clerical and IT/database support. A funding body may be aware that an applicant has core support, so it is important not to overestimate the costs on the grant.

Researchers without access to such resources, who have to be completely self-sufficient, often have to include all costs in the grant application. Although this may make some applications appear to be less financially competitive than others, it is important to be realistic about how much a study will cost. It could be made clear in the application whether core resources are available or not. If they are, applicants could briefly summarise how they could be used to help support the study.

If funding is requested from governmental or charitable organisations, it is good practice to use core resources wherever possible. However, if funding for an academic-led and academic-sponsored study comes from a commercial company, the full cost of the study, including set-up and follow-up, is usually expected to be covered by the grant, as it is likely to be less than the cost incurred if the company conducted the study itself.

6.6 Consideration of costs not to be met by the funding body

The funding body will specify what costs they are or are not willing to meet. If applicants are unsure, administrative staff at the funding organisation can clarify this. Many governmental or charitable organisations will not normally fund the costs of treatments that are already commercially available. There is an expectation that because the manufacturer of a trial treatment (commercial company) will gain from a positive study, they should provide it for free. There may be exceptions to this, for example, where drugs are off-license (off-patent), for example statins or aspirin, in which case a commercial company stands to gain little.

Many studies, particularly clinical trials and cohort studies of humans, incur a *local cost* at the recruiting centre. This could include time spent by local staff involved in the recruitment and management of study participants, and the costs of *extra* clinic assessments, imaging scans, blood tests, pathology reviews, administration of questionnaires, or other evaluations that only arise because of the study (see also Section 6.3). The applicants need to estimate the extent of these expenses, regardless of whether the funding body will support them or not. Local costs will sometimes be considered by the funding committee as part of their evaluation, in addition to, the direct study costs.

A study that has sufficient funds for central co-ordination costs and running expenses could fail in practice because participating centres find the local costs too high and therefore do not take part. To help evaluate the local costs, applicants need to specify the frequency and type of assessments (see also Boxes 4.5 and 4.10). The more additional assessments there are (and the more costly, e.g. CT or PET scans), the more expensive the study, either to the funding body or local service provider. Applicants could therefore try to minimise the number of assessments included in the proposed study.

Occasionally there are clinical trials associated with lower local costs, for example, the test intervention is cheaper or it involves less treatment than the current standard. In this situation it is worth discussing the potential cost-savings in the application, even if they do not affect the amount requested on the grant.

6.7 Grant applications associated with calls for proposals

When there are calls for proposals on the same topic (see Section 1.1.1, page 2), the financial costs are a very important consideration. Applicants are effec-tively in a secret bidding process with each other, and the funding committee should choose the study with the strongest design and methods, but most reasonable costs. While some researchers provide accurate estimates, others may deliberately underestimate costs in order to gain an advantage. This can mean that the study is less likely to finish unless it has access to core resources or, as is more likely, the researchers later request a grant extension. Funding committees may therefore be wary of applications that appear unrealistically inexpensive. Applicants need to be frank about the project costs. If these are properly justified, the funding organisation is likely to accept them. However, it is essential that only necessary items are requested on the grant, without overestimating the level of staff or running expenses required.

6.8 Observational studies in humans (see also Section 4.5, page 44)

When undertaking observational studies on humans, qualitative research studies and case–control studies tend to be less expensive than cohort stud-ies, largely because they do not take as long. The number of staff required will depend on the sample size and anticipated study duration. Almost all observational studies require institutional and/or ethical approval for centres in which subjects will be recruited or where data will be obtained, and the more centres involved, the longer the set-up time, which could be 2–6 months.[3] The set-up time may also need to allow for the development of case report forms (CRFs), questionnaires or interview questions. A CRF is a paper or electronic data sheet that allows the researchers to collect study-specific information about the subjects, including baseline characteristics and details about exposures and lifestyle habits, and disorders. In addition to study set-up time, cohort studies will have a period of follow-up, which can take several years depending on the disorder of interest; common disorders require less follow-up in order to observe a sufficient number of events.

- Qualitative research studies generally involve a relatively small number of subjects, and so may require only a single full-time researcher, or perhaps two or three part-time ones, who would undertake the interviews. Once the interviews are complete, a researcher (often the lead) will need additional time to transcribe and interpret the findings.
- Case–control studies can involve retrospectively collecting data already contained in records (patient files or regional or national datasets), or obtaining it directly from subjects using questionnaires or face-to-face interviews. Many case–control studies use postal questionnaires. Such studies may require a part-time co-ordinator (say 0.5 FTE) throughout if the study is small (e.g. <500 subjects), or a full-time post for a moderate or large study. Depending on the study size and the amount of data that will be entered, this post could also be supported by a clerical/data manager (either part or full time) to help with the mailing of questionnaires and data entry. Consideration should be given to whether data management should be requested for the entire duration of the study, or only part of it.
- Cohort studies require staff to:
  - approach and set up centres from which subjects would be recruited;
  - identify subjects, and possibly arrange baseline assessments, which might include administering questionnaires and/or clinical examinations;
  - arrange the follow-up assessments over subsequent years;
  - respond to any queries from centres or subjects.

All of this work normally requires at least one full-time co-ordinator, and there may also be several research assistants (perhaps part time) spread throughout a geographical region to help with the recruitment and/or study conduct for large projects. As with case–control studies, data management support may also be needed for data entry (0.5 FTE for small studies, or at least one 1.0 FTE for large studies). Occasionally, the statistician or epidemiologist will manage the data, as well as analyse it.

---

[3]In some countries, including the United Kingdom, multicentre studies require national ethical approval, as well as local approval from each recruiting centre.

At least one clerical/data manager position may be needed when there is a significant amount of data from paper CRFs to enter onto a central database within the host institution. However, some case–control or cohort studies involve retrieving data from electronic records held at hospitals, general practice clinics, or from regional or national registries and datasets. These data could be stored in different database formats, so the grant application may need to include a suitably qualified database/IT programmer, who is able to retrieve and collate the data into a single dataset for later analysis. This could be time consuming, depending on the quality of the data sources and whether they contain records in old electronic systems. In such cases, the applicants should request funding for a full-time IT position (1.0 FTE) for at least a year. If all the data are available electronically, the study may only need limited data management support, if at all, and the applicants just request a part- or full-time study co-ordinator (depending on the workload) and a full-time IT post.

Statistical support will also be required, but unless the Study Team intends to conduct analyses during the study, the main statistical analysis will be at the end, and a full-time statistician is probably needed for the last 3–12 months of the grant. During this period, he/she may also raise data queries that have to be checked with the source data, and allowance should be made for this. When applicants do not have access to core resources, it is advisable to request the study co-ordinator for an extra 3 or more months to undertake set-up and obtain all the necessary approvals. Most of the running expenses should be for printing and posting questionnaires (when used), the cost of staff travel to recruiting centres, and occasionally for study subjects to attend for interviews or assessments.

6.8.1 An example

An example of a costing breakdown for a hypothetical cohort study is shown in Table 6.2. The costs assume that there is no access to core resources, and they come from a university financial algorithm. The study is based on 1000 subjects to be recruited from 25 centres; 3 months to set up the study (Year 1, October–December), 2 years of recruitment (Years 2–3, January–December), and 18 months of follow-up (Years 4–5).[4] Data chasing and statistical analysis would occur in the last 6 months of Year 5. All staff costs include salary on-costs and yearly increases within the salary range (including London Weighting), but annual inflation has not been added to the running expenses. Staff costs were approximately the middle of each salary grade (range).

---

[4] The dates are specified in this way so that each staff cost can be seen more easily in each year (considered to be January–December); Year 1 is therefore just an additional 3 months for set-up activities.

Table 6.2 Example of a costing breakdown for a hypothetical cohort study (1000 subjects from 25 recruiting centres)

	Year 1 (Oct–Dec)	Year 2 (Jan–Dec)	Year 3	Year 4	Year 5	
Staff costs						
Research fellow	£11,159	£45,551	£48,694	£52,061	£55,664	
Grade 7	1.0 FTE	1.0 FTE	1.0 FTE	1.0 FTE	1.0 FTE	
IT support	£4,376	£1,786	£1,908	£2,040	£2,154	
Grade 6	0.5 FTE	0.05 FTE	0.05 FTE	0.05 FTE	0.05 FTE	
Data entry	–	–	£3,715	£3,970	£4,242	
Grade 6			0.1 FTE	0.1 FTE	0.1 FTE	
Running expenses						
Office costs (eg printing)	£1,000	£6,000	£6,000	£6,000	£6,000	
Collection & storage of baseline blood samples (£15 per subject)	–	£7,500 (for 500 subjects)	£7,500 (for 500 subjects)	–	–	
Travel for Study Team (5 members, £150 each)	£750	£750	£750	£750	£750	
One-off costs						
Statistical analysis	–	–	–	–	£10,000	
1 personal computer	£500	–	–	–	–	
Software licenses	£500	–	–	–	–	
						Total
Total direct costs	£18,285	£61,587	£68,567	£64,821	£78,810	£292,070
Staff	£15,535	£47,337	£54,317	£58,071	£62,060	£237,320
Other expenses	£2,750	£14,250	£14,250	£6,750	£16,750	£54,750
Indirect costs	£18,254	£75,066	£78,068	£81,194	£84,439	£337,021
Total yearly costs (FECs)	£36,539	£136,653	£146,635	£146,015	£163,249	£629,091

A justification of the costs is as follows:

- A research fellow is needed to oversee (manage) the whole study, as well as provide significant academic/scientific input. This post is needed for 3 months in the first year to set up centres. The research fellow is kept at full time throughout the whole study, but if it were considered that their workload is reduced because of the data management support from Year 3, the post could be reduced to say 0.5 FTE in later years in order to reduce costs.
- In Years 3–5, (recruitment and follow-up), some data management support is included to help with data entry and raising data queries. In Year 2, the amount of data being received may not require additional data management support, and could be undertaken by the research fellow.
- IT support is needed to develop and test the database before the study starts, and then provide support in subsequent years for its maintenance.
- Statistical support is requested only in the final year of the study to develop the analysis programmes, might and conduct the analyses, with input from the Study Team. No planned statistical analyses are intended during the study.
- Running expenses are £6,000 per year once the study starts, which is a reasonable estimate considering that there are 25 recruiting centres, plus the central study co-ordination expenses. A planned translational research sub-study involves obtaining a single blood sample from all study subjects at baseline, at a cost of £15 per subject. The costs do not allow for laboratory storage space, such as a freezer, which would need to be added if required.

The breakdown shows the total costs; they are £629,091 including indirect costs and £292,070 without them. This is equivalent to a cost per subject of £629 or £292 with and without indirect costs. If the Study Team considers them to be too high, or the annual costs exceed that specified by the funding body, savings need to be made, such as removing the translational sub-study or reducing the research fellow staff costs in the later years.

　The type of staff used to manage the project can make a significant difference to the indirect costs. In the example, the data manager, IT post and statistician are all classified as 'service or support', but the research fellow is classified as 'research/academic'. However, if this post were also classified as 'service or support', the indirect costs would be zero (instead of £337,021), even though the same salary range is used (grade 7). This might not seem intuitive, because the same number and grade of staff will be used. The difference is a result of the financial algorithm used, which only attributes indirect costs to academic and research staff and not to support or administrative staff. In the example, it could be decided that someone with an academic background in the field of interest would be more suitable to the post of managing the study than a study co-ordinator, hence the classification of the post. Applicants therefore need to consider carefully which types of roles are appropriate for the study, and whether they are expected to have a research or service support input.

6.9 Clinical trials in humans (see also Section 4.6, page 49)

Because of the need to adhere to regulations and guidelines (see Section 4.6), it can now take several months to set up a multicentre clinical trial. Studies examining an investigational drug must have national regulatory approval in addition to all the other approvals normally required for studies on humans, as well as dealing with contracts and agreements, and developing processes for drug labelling and supply. Applicants often significantly underestimate the time this takes.

If there is no access to core resources (see Section 6.5), applicants could consider adding a trial co-ordinator (or administrative support) to the application for 3–6 months before the trial is expected to actually start recruiting. Otherwise, a member of the Study Team is usually expected to develop and submit all the forms necessary to gain approval to run the trial. For large multicentre studies (national or international), a trial co-ordinator is often essential, because of the significant workload involved.

A clinical trial will encompass many activities:

- Randomising subjects (randomised trials only).
- Dealing with queries from participating centres.
- Implementing and checking systems for drug supply and distribution are in place.
- Making changes to the protocol or other documentation, and then getting these approved by, for example, institutional review boards, ethics committees or regulatory authorities.
- Entering data that comes in on paper CRFs.
- Monitoring safety and adverse events, including receiving and processing serious event notifications, and reporting them to the regulatory authority or other necessary parties.
- Having general oversight of all recruiting centres.

In addition to the conduct of the trial, other activities may be required:

- Statistical analyses during and at the end of the trial.
- Pathology reviews.
- Central reviews of imaging.
- Central laboratory testing of biological samples.
- Health economic assessments.

When necessary, all these have to be included in the grant application, either as staff costs or support costs.

At the end of the trial, part-time data management or clerical support may be needed to close down the study at each centre (say 0.1 FTE for 3 months). This involves ensuring that outstanding major data queries have been resolved, and that centres have all the necessary trial documentation in place before they archive their files into long-term storage.

Small, simple clinical trials to be conducted in only a few centres (e.g. <5, and with <100 subjects) may only require one person to co-ordinate the study and enter the data. This position may not even need to be full time, depending on the complexity of the trial. Larger, multicentre clinical trials, with >100 subjects, often need a full-time co-ordinator, and the number of additional staff will be influenced by the number of centres, whether the proposed trial is to be conducted internationally, and the amount of data to be entered. A 4-year trial of, for example, 500 subjects should be adequately supported by a 1.0 FTE trial co-ordinator and up to one 0.5 FTE data manager, while a 3-year trial of 5000 subjects may require a 1.0 FTE trial co-ordinator and at least one 1.0 FTE data manager.

6.9.1 On-site monitoring

On-site monitoring allows the host institution (i.e. the Sponsor) to have oversight of the trial at participating centres, and to check that the systems in place are appropriate and correctly followed. This could include checking that trial subjects are verified and that data have not been falsified; that the protocol is followed correctly; that drugs are being labelled and distributed correctly; that serious adverse events are being reported and that this is being done within the specified time limits; and that the data recorded on CRFs match those in the original hospital records (called *source data verification*, SDV). Commercially funded and sponsored trials will often have dedicated trial monitors who regularly visit each centre. SDV is an expensive activity, and there is a lack of evidence on whether it is worthwhile in randomised trials. Many trials sponsored and funded within academic institutions have minimal on-site monitoring for phase III trials, and instead may rely on central data checks at the co-ordinating centre, or visits to recruiting centres only when a problem is suspected. However, a commercial company may specifically request full on-site monitoring (for registration and licensing purposes following a positive trial), in addition to a trial co-ordination and data management support, although this increases the costs. For small studies, the trial co-ordinator or data manager may undertake on-site monitoring functions as well as their other tasks, while for larger studies a separate monitor post could be requested (generally 0.5–1.0 FTE, depending on the number of recruiting centres).

Monitoring activities may be appropriate for phase I and II trials, particularly when these involve new and unlicensed therapies, there are expected serious side effects, or the trial includes children or incapacitated or vulnerable adults. One of the main purposes of the monitoring visit is, in these cases, to ensure that the procedures for administering drugs and safety reporting are being followed correctly. Checking source data associated with key variables might also be useful in small early phase trials in order to reduce error and improve the precision of the results.

Applicants should consider how much on-site monitoring is likely to be needed, according to the type of trial being conducted, and ensure that funds are requested to cover this in the grant.

6.9.2 An example

An example of a costing breakdown for a hypothetical placebo-controlled clinical trial of an investigational drug is shown in Table 6.3. The study is based on 500 subjects to be recruited from 30 centres. It is expected that 6 months is needed to set up the study (Year 1); 2 years of recruitment (Years 2–3) and 1 year of follow-up (Year 4); and data chasing, statistical analysis and close-down of the trial in centres in Year 5. Similar to the example in Section 6.8.1, staff costs include salary on-costs and yearly increases.

A justification of the costs is as follows:

- A full-time trial co-ordinator is needed to set up the trial, and manage the study during recruitment and follow-up.
- The part-time data manager is only required after enough data is received regularly (i.e. the last 6 months of Year 2, after recruitment has started, and during follow-up). In the final year, limited data management support (0.1 FTE) is used to close down the trial at centres and chase up any outstanding key data items.
- Both the co-ordinator and data manager are responsible for data entry and data checking (there will be several CRFs per patient), processing serious adverse events, and they could undertake on-site monitoring activities when required.
- The statistician is needed at the start of trial to help develop the CRFs and the method of randomisation, and in subsequent years to conduct interim statistical analyses of recruitment, safety, treatment compliance and efficacy for the IDMC. In the final year, the statistician FTE increases to allow enough time for a full analysis and help with writing the report.
- IT support is needed to develop the randomisation system and database, but once in place there should only need to be limited support to maintain them during the study.

Table 6.3 Example of a costing breakdown for a hypothetical phase III clinical trial of an investigational drug (500 patients from 30 centres)

	Year 1 (July–Dec)	Year 2 (Jan–Dec)	Year 3	Year 4	Year 5 (Jan–June)	
Staff costs						
Study co-ordinator Grade 7	£22,173 1.0 FTE	£45,551 1.0 FTE	£48,694 1.0 FTE	£52,061 1.0 FTE	– –	
Statistician Grade 7	£1,135 0.05 FTE	£2,341 0.05 FTE	£2,503 0.05 FTE	£2,676 0.05 FTE	£27,579 1.0 FTE	
IT support Grade 7	£5,579 0.5 FTE (3 months)	£456 0.01 FTE	£487 0.01 FTE	£521 0.01 FTE	£268 0.01 FTE	
Data manager Grade 6	– –	£9,251 0.5 FTE (last 6 months)	£19,085 0.5 FTE	£20,395 0.5 FTE	£2,101 0.1 FTE	
Running expenses						
Printing, postage, stationery, etc.	£1,000	£3,000	£3,000	£3,000	£1,000	
Regulatory agency fees	£4,500	£400	£400	£400	£400	
Travel for Study Team (5 members, £150 each)	£750	£750	£750	£750	£750	
Travel for IDMC (3 members, £150 each)	£450	£450	£450	£450	–	
One-off costs						
2 personal computers	£1,000	–	–	–	–	
Software licenses	£1,000	–	–	–	–	
Health economics	£10,000	–	–	–	–	
						Total
Total direct costs	£47,587	£62,199	£75,369	£80,253	£32,098	*£297,506*
Staff	£28,887	£57,599	£70,769	£75,653	£29,948	£262,856
Other expenses	£18,700	£4,600	£4,600	£4,600	£2,150	£34,650
*Indirect costs**	£2,045	£4,186	£4,353	£4,527	£2,311	*£17,422*
Total yearly costs (FECs)	£49,632	£66,385	£79,722	£84,780	£34,409	*£314,928*

*Includes the cost of the time spent on the project by a co-applicant (1 hour per week) who is based in the host institution.

- All trials of an investigational drug must obtain national regulatory approval (e.g. from the Competent Authority in Europe, or the Food and Drug Administration in the United States), and this usually incurs an initial application cost, and sometimes a modest annual cost while the study is being conducted.
- As well as meetings of the Study Team, the IDMC also need to meet, in this example a year after the trial has started, and annually thereafter.
- An one-off cost is a health economist who would spend perhaps 3 months to perform a cost-effectiveness analysis.

A breakdown of the costs is shown in Table 6.3, and is interpreted in a similar way as that for the cohort study example in Section 6.8.1. All the staff posts are classified as service support and not academic/research, hence the indirect costs are relatively low (they are based only on input from a senior academic based in the host institution who is a co-applicant on the grant). The total direct costs are £297,506, which is reasonable for a study of this size and duration. Other trials may require, for example, more data management support, data monitors or dedicated administrative support, depending on the complexity of the study.

6.10 Laboratory experiments (see also Section 4.7, page 57)

The types of staff requested on a grant application associated with a laboratory experiment are different from those for observational studies or clinical trials of humans. Staff are normally only required in the laboratory and can be one or more of the following full-time (1.0 FTE) employees:

- Laboratory technician.
- Research technician.
- Postdoctoral research fellow.
- Clinical research fellow.
- Scientist/senior scientist.

The number and type of each post required will depend on the complexity and scope of the proposed experiment, for example, there could be several distinct but related stages, and one person would work on each stage. Applicants should also check whether all staff categories would have associated indirect costs. For example, a laboratory technician post (who may undertake routine tests as part of the proposed experiment or just be involved in preparing/storing samples) may not be eligible for indirect costs, but a research technician post (who may be responsible for developing a new method/technique for the experiment, such as finding new ways of extracting DNA) could have indirect costs added.

A significant proportion of the grant may also be required to cover equipment, reagents and other materials, necessary to conduct the experiment. These costs should be estimated carefully using published list prices or quotes from commercial companies, though researchers should try to get an academic discount for some of the costs. There may also be costs arising from purchasing and maintaining animals, license fees, or for implementing safety procedures to protect staff from hazardous substances or exposures. Materials to be purchased each year would be considered as running expenses, while equipment would normally be classified as a one-off expense.

Expensive or highly specialised laboratory equipment usually have a warranty (for yearly maintenance and breakdown), at an annual cost. This could be as much as £10,000 or more per year, and applicants should ensure that this is added to the application. Sometimes, other research groups in the host institution may be able to use the equipment, so it might be more efficient to spread the purchase and warranty cost between several groups (and several grant applications if possible). Funding bodies sometimes have an upper limit for a single piece of equipment, and applicants should consult administrative staff at the funding if the cost is likely to exceed this.

The approach to estimating costs in laboratory experiments is similar to that in Tables 6.2 and 6.3, but with different categories of staff, and with a detailed breakdown of the key materials, animals and equipment to be used.

6.11 Systematic reviews (see also Section 4.10, page 69)

Funding bodies have a general preference to provide grants for large systematic reviews, which involve the collection, assimilation and analysis of many published studies, or for retrieving the raw data from each of the several research groups that conducted the original study. This usually requires a full-time research assistant, who would be supervised by the Study Team over 1–2 years. The appointed person will have to conduct a thorough search of the published medical literature to identify potential studies, obtain the full text of those articles that are relevant to the review, extract information from each article, write to the research team of each study to request the raw data (for an Individual Patient Data systematic review), retrieve and collate the data, and raise any queries with the original research team. In addition to funding for the research assistant, other items on the grant application may include:

- Obtaining hard copies of all the papers identified from the literature search that appear to be relevant (this could cost up to £5 per paper, and a review could have between 10 and over a 100 studies).

- Statistical support to conduct the meta-analysis at the end (e.g. a full-time statistician for 6 months). This may or may not be part of the role of the person who conducted the review.
- Travel for members of each research group who provided raw data to meet and discuss the findings of the systematic review.
- A modest fee to each study group (e.g. £200 per study) to cover the cost of the time preparing the dataset, and labelling and defining all the variables requested, because this can take up to two days (especially if the data are kept in an old database system, and needs cleaning). However, this may be too expensive if there are many studies to include in the review.

Summary points

- Do not request excessive costs that are clearly not justified by the study design.
- Do not request too many staff on the grant, especially if the proposed study is relatively small, or large amounts of data are not expected.
- When estimating staff costs ensure that all relevant add-on costs are included, not just the salary to the post-holder.
- Fully justify each major cost item.
- Do not underestimate the costs of study set-up and conduct.
- Check with the host institution and funding body whether indirect costs (overheads) need to be estimated and added to the grant.
- Use core resources, where possible, for some study activities.

Chapter 7 **Funding body review process**

Chapters 3–5 have concentrated on the grant application itself and other associated documents. It is also worth understanding what the review process entails, including the covering letter, external reviewers and how the project proposal is likely to be evaluated by the funding committee. This knowledge could influence the contents of the application.

7.1 Submitting the application

Applicants spend most of their time on the grant application contents, but there are two other important aspects of the submission: the covering letter, and who to nominate as the external reviewers.

7.1.1 Covering letter

All applications should be accompanied by a covering letter. It provides the funding body committee and the external reviewers with the most important points of the proposed study. This should not include details of the study but rather one or two <u>short</u> paragraphs covering:

- The primary objective.
- The value of the study.
- How the results and conclusions could be used.

The covering letter should fit onto a single page; overly verbose letters are unnecessary. The application form will almost always have space for an abstract, and there will be several sections within which to provide details about the study, so there is no need to repeat this information in the covering letter.

How to Write a Grant Application, 1st edition. © Allan Hackshaw. Published 2011 by Blackwell Publishing Ltd.

7.1.2 Nominating external reviewers

Many funding bodies send the application to external *reviewers* (*referees*) for comment. The reviewers are experts in the field and will be able to provide constructive comments on the application in relation to:

- Feasibility.
- The likely impact or value of the study.
- Possible design flaws.
- Competing studies.
- Likelihood of completing on time.

These comments are used by the funding committee to help them decide whether to approve the project or not, and the applicants are not usually informed of the names of the reviewers.[1] However, some funding bodies operate an open review system in which the names of the external reviewers are provided to the applicants, and there are both advantages and disadvantages to this. An advantage is that there is a degree of openness, so that an applicant would be made aware of a reviewer with a bias or conflict of interest. A disadvantage is that reviewers may be less inclined to be honest about their opinions on the application in order to avoid creating a professional rivalry.

The applicants can recommend external reviewers on the application form, though the funding body is under no obligation to use these nominations. The suggested reviewers should not be in the same institution as the chief investigator, or have any direct involvement in the proposed study. The reviewers are often well-known experts in the field, but sometimes they are professional colleagues of one or more members of the Study Team. They must be chosen carefully, on the basis of their expertise and ability to provide sensible and unbiased comments. A professional colleague should not be suggested simply because of a previous working (and friendly) relationship, because it might be a mistake to assume that they will only give positive and supportive comments. If the study design is not of a high standard or is scientifically flawed, or the application is poorly written, the external reviewer could be in a difficult predicament; caught between being honest with their comments, or supportive of a colleague. Usually, his/her own professional reputation comes first, in that it would be inappropriate to give unwarranted praise, knowing that there will be other reviewers.

Occasionally, there is a section in the application where applicants have the opportunity to list people who they prefer *not* to be used as an external reviewer. The section should only be completed if there are individuals who

---

[1] In the same way that referees of papers submitted for publication to journals are usually kept anonymous.

are likely to provide a biased or unfair assessment. This may occur if, for example, the proposed study competes with work of the reviewer, or if there has been a previous professional rivalry. Applicants should provide only a few names, if necessary, and not a long list.

7.2 Processing the application within the funding body

The administrative staff at the funding body will have quite strict deadlines to work towards, and will be dealing with multiple applications. They need to:

- Process the applications internally, including logging them onto an internal database, and checking that the required documents have been received and the relevant signatures obtained.
- Identify appropriate external reviewers and send the application to them; this may involve making many photocopies and posting a hard copy to each reviewer (if not done by email).
- Receive and process the reviewers' comments and, when relevant, send them out to the applicants.
- Receive the response from applicants, and process them in time for the funding committee meeting, ensuring that all committee members have the full grant submissions, external reviewers' comments and applicants' responses.

Often, only a few staff dealing with many applications have to do all of this.

After the funding committee has met, it usually takes at least 3 weeks before the applicant receives feedback. It can be a tense time because a researcher's employment or career could depend on successful funding. In order to understand why this process takes so long, it is useful to know the course of action that follows the meeting. The minutes or notes for each application taken during the meeting need to be written up by the administrative staff and used to draft the feedback for applicants. These comments are then reviewed and edited by at least one committee member. Sometimes, the three or four members who were assigned the project proposal will be involved in drafting the feedback which is often reviewed and approved by the committee Chair, or delegate. All of these activities take time, whether correspondence is by post or email, because the people involved will be based at different institutions.

7.3 Initial reviews (external reviewers)

If a funding organisation has sent the application to external reviewers, the comments are sometimes forwarded to the applicants for a response, before the committee meets.[2] This allows the applicants a chance to address any concerns raised and to clarify any misunderstandings. Usually, the applicants do not need to edit and resubmit the application form; all that is required is a response to the comments.

It is possible to form a *preliminary* view on the level of interest at this stage, but it would be erroneous to interpret positive comments as a guarantee to success, or to presume negative comments will lead to rejection, because the committee that makes the final decision has not met yet. However, this is an important opportunity for the applicants to improve the chance of being funded. It is very common to receive both positive and negative comments, and there are occasions when at least one of the reviewers has misinterpreted part of the application, not read it in sufficient detail, or where their comments do not appear to be clear or constructive. In such circumstances, the response from the applicants must not be dismissive, or give any impression of being annoyed by the comments made. More often than not, there is a genuine misunderstanding by a reviewer which was due to a lack of clarity in the application, or they are interested in details omitted from the application due to lack of space.

There are many occasions when the list of comments looks so daunting at first that the applicants believe the study proposal has already failed. However, often after reading through the comments carefully, the situation is far less severe than it first appears and the comments are relatively easy to deal with. It is important to remain calm and focussed, and to deal with each issue raised.

There are several useful points to bear in mind when replying to the reviewers' comments:

- It is helpful to assign numbers to the comments if they are not already numbered, and include these in the response that will be examined by the funding committee. This will make it easier for the funding committee to match each response to the original comment. Alternatively, each response could start with some brief keywords (underlined or in italics) that are associated with the comment being addressed. For example, if a reviewer questioned the sample size calculation, the response could start with:
  - '*Sample size: Our justification for the sample size estimate was based on published references and consensus between the investigators …*'
- Avoid pasting all of the original comments into the response and putting the reply underneath each one. This is unnecessary and makes the document significantly longer. Some applicants believe this approach makes it easier to match a response to a reviewer's comment, but a good response will indicate

---

[2] All funding bodies should do this, but unfortunately this is not the case.

what the original comment was. There is no need to send the funding committee the original reviewers' comments when they already have them.

- Each comment should be taken in turn and addressed as concisely as possible. A long, rambling response could give the funding committee the impression that the applicants are not clear enough about their own study, or that they are trying to avoid providing a direct answer. Short responses could indicate that the comments and criticisms were relatively easy to deal with, and this might strengthen the application.

- Some comments clearly do not require a response, so the applicants may not need to address them. However, if the comment or statement made is very positive, or is relevant to something raised by another reviewer, it could be mentioned in the response.

- Be careful about the tone of language – try to be helpful and positive throughout the response, and not antagonistic, condescending or defensive. Therefore, try to avoid words such as 'simply', 'clearly' or 'obviously'. If unsure, it might be worth showing the response to a colleague who is not involved in the project.

- If the applicant agrees with a reviewer's comment, then it might be appropriate to discuss how the proposed project would change because of it. This might involve a change to the study design (e.g. different outcome measures, a lower or greater sample size, or having different methods).

- If the applicant disagrees with a comment, then the response should be properly justified, preferably with published references or other factual evidence, rather than personal opinion. If the comment was due to some misinterpretation of a section in the form, the applicants should explain what they meant in a different way, and not reiterate or repeat what was in the original application.

- If two or more reviewers make the same comment, this is probably a sign of something important, and so should definitely be addressed properly.

- If one reviewer contradicts another, then applicants must themselves choose the one that is more appropriate, and it is helpful to note the inconsistency and justify the choice.

- All the reviewers' comments that require a response should be addressed. Ignoring a response will not weaken the reviewer's criticism, and may instead draw further attention and interest to the point.

It should be noted that the external reviewers' comments are not usually the deciding factor in determining the success of an application, but rather they contribute to the committee's final decision. Therefore, it is possible that even if all the reviewers are generally supportive, the application could be rejected. Similarly, even if the comments are generally negative, the application could still be successful.

7.4 Funding committee meeting

The funding committee, often 10–20 people, will include several experts, usually with different scientific backgrounds in order to provide a comprehensive assessment of each application. They will make the decision to fund a project or not. All applications, external reviewers' comments and applicants' response to these comments (when available) are sent to the committee several weeks before the meeting to allow members sufficient time to read and assess all the material.

For governmental, academic or charitable funding organisations, members would have been invited onto the committee in recognition of their expertise, or they may have applied to be a member through competitive selection. Such individuals tend to come from academic institutions or hospitals. Within a commercial organisation, the funding committee is usually an internal Scientific Board, composed of senior staff who work for the company and sometimes external advisors.

The frequency of the funding committee meetings will vary according to the organisation. Larger organisations tend to meet perhaps three or four times each year, while smaller ones may only convene annually. When there are specific calls for study proposals, there could be a dedicated meeting. Commercial company scientific boards could meet as often as monthly.

The format of the meetings will also vary according to the organisation. If there are relatively few applications, all the committee members may be expected to read through and comment on all applications. However, larger organisations could have as many as 50 or more applications to be considered at a single meeting. Because it can take at least 2 hours to properly evaluate an application, it would be unreasonable to expect each member to evaluate every application in detail. Therefore, the workload may be spread across the committee so that each application is assigned to about three or four members. These individuals will review the application closely, consider the external reviewers' comments and determine whether they are valid or not, and whether these comments have been satisfactorily addressed by the applicants (when available). The other committee members are still expected to look through all the other applications that they were not specifically assigned, but not in as much detail.

If a member of the committee is part of the proposed study, either as a co-investigator or collaborator, or they work in the same department as the lead applicant, they should not be involved in the decision-making process, and are usually required to leave the room when the application is being discussed. Members are obliged to state any potential conflict of interest associated with any application.

During the meeting, the group of three or four members assigned specifically to evaluate a particular application will each give their opinions on the proposed study to the full committee, after which follows a discussion on the strengths and limitations of the proposal. Otherwise, all members provide their assessment. Longer discussions tend to be associated with large and expensive studies, or those with significant problems. It is common for some members to be supportive of an application and others not, so one of the main purposes of the discussion is to try to get a consensus. At the end, the Chair will usually summarise the views of the committee. A unanimous decision is then generally reached on whether or not a project should be funded, perhaps conditional on further clarifications or changes to the study from the applicants. In the unlikely event of not having a consensus, the Chair may make the final decision. Sometimes, the applicants are invited to resubmit a revised application to the next committee meeting (if possible), after addressing the concerns of the members who had criticisms.

Some funding bodies assign a numerical score to each application, derived from scores provided by each committee member (e.g. the average). The scoring range differs depending on the funding organisation. For example, the Medical Research Council (United Kingdom) and Cancer Research UK use a range of 0–10 (10 is the best score), while the US National Institutes of Health uses 100–500 (100 is the best score). The funding organisation will then use this score to determine which projects are funded or not. They may take only those in the highest pre-specified centile (e.g. top 10%), or there could be a threshold score above which there is an obligation to fund all applications. If either of these is the approach of the funding body, applicants need to aim to obtain a high rank for their project when writing the application (see next section). Furthermore, the score given by each committee member is likely to be correlated with the scores given by the three or four members who evaluated the application in detail.

7.5 Funding committee evaluation

During the committee meeting, the discussions will focus on several aspects of the application, which together influence the final decision (Figure 7.1). The more of these aspects that are addressed in the background and justification for the study, and study design, the more likely that it would score highly and receive funding.

7.5.1 Innovation

The committee will determine whether the proposed study is new (i.e. has never been done before); uses novel experimental or laboratory techniques;

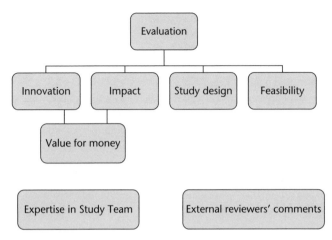

Figure 7.1 Key aspects of a grant application used by a funding committee for evaluation purposes.

or uses a novel design or statistical methods (see also Section 3.6, page 31). However, there should be nothing wrong with repeating a study that has been done elsewhere, possibly in a different country or among a different subgroup of individuals. In fact, having two or more studies on the same subject that yield similar results greatly increases the justification for changing practice. Similarly, it may show reproducibility in an experimental study, making the conclusions more reliable. Committee members are normally aware of what other evidence is available or which comparable or similar studies are in progress, so they will determine what the proposed study could add to these.

7.5.2 Impact – the importance of the research
Impact is related to innovation (see previous section), but is not necessarily the same. Some studies may not be considered particularly innovative but could potentially have a large impact on practice. There are several reasons why a proposed project would be useful, for example, the result may:
- Change clinical practice with regard to prevention, diagnosis or treatment, or improving patients' quality of life – for example, a new intervention is introduced, or it becomes more commonly used (i.e. the standard).
- Influence public health education – for example, identifying newly identified risk factors for disorders or early death, or recommend lifestyle habits that can benefit physical or psychological health.
- Add to current knowledge about people's characteristics, attitude or behaviour – for example, finding out how many people exercise regularly.

- Add to current scientific knowledge, such as biological, pharmacological, physiological or psychological mechanisms – for example, a better understanding of how a disease is caused or progresses, or is treated.
- Help to design further and larger studies – for example, using positive results from a phase II clinical trial to design a phase III trial.

There is sometimes a misconception that only studies that change clinical practice are funded, but this is not necessarily the case. There are many projects that provide useful new information on a specific field of research, or will lead to other studies that will themselves influence practice. It is important to make clear in the application why the proposed study is needed. The external reviewers and funding committee will form their own opinions on the impact, but it is something that has a significant influence on the decision on whether to fund the study.

7.5.3 Value for money

All funding organisations, even those that are considered wealthy, have limited funds. The committee will therefore often seek to balance the financial costs of the project against innovation, and particularly impact. Impact is probably more important to many funding bodies (particularly for charitable organisations or foundations), because they can use the results and conclusions of a study[3] in their public relations and marketing campaigns, which in turn can help raise funds to be invested back into research. A small but expensive study, with minimal impact, is unlikely to be funded, even if it has some novel aspect. Similarly, a single large study that could have a potentially moderate impact might not be successful if it were very expensive, because funding it could mean that two or more cheaper studies that could also have a moderate impact are not funded.

Evaluating whether a particular study proposal could be value for money is difficult. It may also depend on the strategic policies of the funding organisation, and the projected funds available in a given year. When a scoring system and threshold is used, considering value for money is easier because the score is largely based on scientific merit and impact. As long as these are met and the application exceeds the threshold, it would normally be funded. However, when there are calls for proposals on a specific topic, only a single study can be selected and value for money is a key determining factor.

Although the funding committee will comment on the financial costs requested in an application, and the costs may influence their decision, it is ultimately up to the funding organisation (represented by senior administrative staff at the committee meeting) to determine whether it can afford a

---

[3] Particularly if these lead to a change in clinical or public health practice.

particular project or not. A strong project proposal that is too expensive may be sent back to the applicants with a request to reduce costs. Occasionally, an overly expensive study is rejected on this basis alone.

7.5.4 Strong scientific design

Most grant application forms have been specifically designed to bring out the most important aspects of the proposed study in relation to the objectives and study design. The funding committee will determine whether:

- The most appropriate design is used.
- The most appropriate outcome measures are used, particularly the primary endpoint(s).
- The sample size estimate is acceptable (and not overly small or large), and that it is correct (a statistical reviewer will often try to replicate the estimate using information provided in the application).
- There are any important biases in the study design that have not been addressed and minimised.
- There are any scientific flaws in the way subjects for the study (or biological samples) are selected, managed or treated, and how the endpoints are obtained or measured.
- Important potential confounding factors are adequately considered (observational studies).
- The statistical methods of analysis are appropriate.

Considering and addressing all of the above satisfactorily when developing the grant application should increase the chance of success; however, this can only be done if the description of the study design is sufficiently clear.

7.5.5 Feasibility and likelihood of completion in a reasonable timescale

Many researchers underestimate the work required to set up and conduct studies, especially large-scale surveys, case–control and cohort studies, and clinical trials. A funding body will expect that a study is completed on time, or not long after. Therefore, if there is a high chance that the study duration would be significantly extended, it may be difficult to successfully obtain funding.

For many studies, two of the most important aspects are to recruit enough subjects and to obtain the main outcome measures on all (or most) of them. Studies can fail because:

- Not enough centres (from which study subjects would be recruited) actually take part, even though some showed initial interest at the time of the grant application.
- There are far fewer eligible subjects than originally anticipated.

- There are far fewer eligible subjects who wish to participate, for example, they do not want to be allocated to one of the interventions in a particular randomised clinical trial (subjects find them too invasive, or they already have a preference for one of the trial treatments).
- Many subjects decline to participate or they initially agree but later drop out because there are too many or too frequent assessments (or they are too invasive), so the outcome measures cannot be obtained on enough subjects for a reliable analysis.
- The local financial costs incurred as a direct result of conducting a study in humans are so high that few centres will actually participate (see Section 6.6, page 87); this could also be due to having too many or too frequent assessments.
- The study duration is so long that newer interventions, technologies or laboratory methods are likely to supersede those used in the project, making the study objectives irrelevant or obsolete.
- A laboratory experiment is based on methods that are too labour intensive, or the project is too complex (e.g. too many hypotheses).

Feasibility is more of a problem with studies of humans, so it is important to discuss potential recruitment in the application (see Section 3.5, page 29, feasibility). Even if the study idea is novel and highly interesting, it could fail on the basis of a high likelihood that not enough subjects would take part. Applicants should therefore attempt to provide some evidence that the study is likely to be feasible.

7.5.6 Sufficient expertise in the Study Team

Most projects require multiple areas of expertise, so the committee will want to see that all of these are represented in the proposed project, ideally by suitably experienced co-investigators or collaborators (see Box 2.2 on page 18 for examples). Applications[4] that come from only one or two co-applicants, and there are no named collaborators, could be viewed negatively, because it can indicate a lack of general support for the study, or one that has not been thought through properly. A group of applicants with hardly any previous work in the proposed project is unlikely to be funded, even if the individual members are highly experienced in other fields. A chief investigator with a solid history of research publications, previous successful grant applications or a good track record of finishing studies on time will probably have a better chance of success than someone who is new to research. Therefore, a researcher who is at the start of their career should endeavour to work with some more experienced co-applicants. This is less important for applications

---

[4] Usually not training fellowships or doctoral research studentships.

associated with funding for doctoral degrees or training fellowships, which are specifically aimed at new researchers.

7.5.7 External reviewers' comments

The committee will judge whether there is general support from the external reviewers, and that any criticism or potential problems they have raised have been adequately addressed by the applicants, including recommended changes to the study design (see Section 7.3).

7.6 Feedback to applicants after the meeting

After the funding committee has met, the feedback is sent to applicants by post and/or email, with one of several decisions depending on the policies within the funding organisation and the type of grant being applied for:

- Successful – no changes required.
- Successful – but conditional on minor or major changes or clarifications.
- Subject is of interest, but major revisions to the application are required. Applicants are invited to revise and resubmit to the next committee meeting (this may not occur when there are specific calls for proposals).
- Rejection.

If the application is to be reconsidered after major revisions, or is rejected, the reasons for this should be clearly stated in the feedback letter. It is important that the applicants should not take the criticisms personally, but rather read through them carefully to see how the application could be improved, either for resubmission to the same funding body or to another. If an application is rejected, the researchers should not necessarily assume that the proposed project was uninteresting or scientifically poor. It could simply mean that it did not rank highly enough in relation to all the other applications considered at the time. All funding bodies have limited funds, so it is common even for good applications to be unsuccessful.

Some funding organisations are more encouraging to researchers than others, so the option of resubmitting to the next committee meeting is used instead of an outright rejection. There is no guarantee that if all the recommended changes are made that the application will be successful. However, it does give the applicants one more chance.

The decision to reject is almost always based on scientific merit, strength of study design and financial costs. There are occasions when unfortunately the decision has been influenced by political or personal factors, but this is rare and difficult, if not impossible, to prove. Even if an applicant believes this to be the case, they should consider carefully the ramifications of challenging the funding body. Such a challenge is unlikely to be successful and will almost inevitably reflect badly on the applicant.

Occasionally, the funding committee is highly supportive of a project proposal but consider that the financial costs requested are too high. The feedback letter may therefore ask the applicants to reduce the costs, sometimes by specifying which items (i.e. staff or other expenses) might be adjusted. Committee members and administrative staff have significant knowledge and experience in the subject area, and will therefore have a realistic idea of how much a certain study should cost.

7.7 Responding to the funding committee feedback

Unless specifically requested, no response is required after the feedback. If the application has been successful but conditional on relatively minor changes or clarification, the applicants should not automatically presume that funding has been approved. Although the comments may be considered minor, they are clearly important enough to the committee to delay giving a final decision. These comments should be treated in the same way as the initial external reviewers' comments (see Section 7.3), and a response should be sent back to the funding body as soon as possible. If the applicants have been asked to reduce the costs, they should try to do so as much as possible. If there are areas in which it really would be inappropriate to do so without affecting the scientific integrity of the study, the applicants should defend their position very clearly in the feedback letter. It is often helpful to speak to the administrative staff at the funding body about costs before responding to the committee. The applicants' response is usually reviewed by only one or two members of the committee and the Chair (*Chairman's action*), and the final decision is sent shortly afterwards.

If the application has been deferred to the next meeting, it usually means that major changes are required, usually to the design (e.g. outcome measures, or methods), or insufficient prior evidence was given. The fact that the proposal has not been rejected outright indicates that the funding committee is interested in the project, so applicants should ensure that the criticisms and recommendations have been dealt with satisfactorily. A revised application form is expected to be submitted by the deadline for the next committee meeting; applicants are not required to respond immediately. The feedback letter from the committee should be clear about the necessary revisions, and the applicants should ensure that these are all made. If there is a disagreement in relation to one or more of the comments, the applicants should justify their position carefully, preferably with reference to the literature. Occasionally, all of the recommended changes are inappropriate so the applicants may wish to consider whether to wait until the next meeting to respond (which could be several months away), or to do so now.[5] Applicants should first check with the administrative staff at the funding body to determine whether this is possible, but the reasons must be solid and completely defendable. One of the senior committee members or Chair may make an assessment of the situation, but it is difficult to overturn the initial decision without referring the matter for discussion by the whole committee.

When an application is rejected, it usually means that there is no chance of revising and resubmitting it. The reasons are likely to be associated with aspects covered in Section 7.5. Many funding bodies are clear about rejections, and may stipulate that the committee's decision is final. This means that there are not normally grounds for an *appeal*, where the applicants attempt to change the decision. To appeal in this situation should only be done when there are *major factual errors* made by the committee in evaluating the application that had a clear bearing on the decision to reject. A hypothetical example could be where the funding committee believed that the most appropriate study design is different to that proposed by the applicants (e.g. a clinical trial instead of an observational study), but in fact the committee's choice is scientifically flawed. If something like this has occurred, the applicants could consider appealing even if the funding organisation does not normally allow it. Funding committees occasionally make mistakes, and therefore should be made aware if it is likely to have happened. The funding body may then decide that the application can be discussed at the next committee meeting, which is not ideal but at least there is now a chance of funding. An appeal should not be made on the basis of only a difference of opinion with the funding committee. This could irritate the committee, and highly unlikely to overturn the initial decision.

Summary points

- Send a clear, single-page covering letter with the application form that provides a very brief overview of the importance of the proposed study, and its main objective or hypothesis.
- When required, nominate sensible external reviewers.
- When available, read the initial external reviewers' comments carefully and aim to provide a brief, factual and unemotional response to each one.

---

[5] This matters when someone's employment is reliant on the funding being made available soon.

- Bear in mind what the funding committee will look for in an application, namely originality or innovation, potential impact on knowledge or practice, strong study design, evidence of feasibility, sufficient expertise within the Study Team and support from the external reviewers' comments.
- If revisions are required, ensure that these are done as soon as possible, or in time for the next funding committee meeting.
- Do not appeal after an application has been rejected unless absolutely justified, and is based on a substantial factual error made by the funding committee.
- If an application is rejected, carefully consider the reasons why, and revise the study design accordingly before submitting to another funding body.

Chapter 8 **Annual reports and applying for a grant extension**

If a grant application is successful, the researchers may be expected to continually update the funding body during the project, usually every year. Sometimes, it will be clear that the study cannot complete on time, or circumstances change which means that the study must be extended. The researchers may then have to apply for a grant extension. Researchers should be aware that although a grant has been awarded for a specific project, the funding body can terminate it early at any time; it does not have to be automatically renewed each year. This could be after an unfavourable annual report has been received, the study may have already answered its research question, or a grant extension application is declined.

8.1 Annual reports

Many funding organisations require annual reports from the researchers,[1] while others may only request brief information about the study's progress periodically. This allows them to monitor general progress and be informed of any major changes to the study design or conduct, or whether there are any problems that are likely to have a significant impact on the project. Substantial changes to the design may need approval from the funding committee before they can be implemented, especially if they have a direct impact on the primary objectives. An example is when the target sample size has been significantly reduced or increased compared with that specified in the original grant application.

---

[1] This is usual for large funding bodies.

How to Write a Grant Application, 1st edition. © Allan Hackshaw. Published 2011 by Blackwell Publishing Ltd.

A funding body will either have an annual report form for researchers to complete, or specify what information is required. Such reports tend to be relatively concise (e.g. two to five pages), and could show the following:

- Which milestones have been completed, and the current stage of the project.
- For cohort studies or clinical trials of humans, state how many subjects have been recruited so far, the monthly or quarterly accrual rate since the study began, and the total number of activated centres. In a table, list the names of all the activated centres, and indicate the date when each was open to recruitment, the dates of the first and the last recruited subject, and the number per centre. The names of centres being set up could be listed in another table, perhaps with some brief comment on the current status of each, and when activation is likely to occur. It is also useful to say how many other centres have shown interest but have not yet started the set up process.
- How much money has been spent, and on what (with a focus on staff costs).

The researchers should highlight what they consider to be key achievements. The report could be reviewed at the next funding committee meeting or internally by administrative staff within the funding organisation, and the grant will usually be renewed for the following year if there are no substantial concerns.

If there are major problems, or changes to the primary objectives or design, the researchers will need to describe and justify these clearly in the annual report, though in some circumstances the funding body should be informed sooner than this. More importantly, the Study Team needs to explain how they propose to solve any problems in the forthcoming months. These details are required in addition to information on milestones, current status and costs incurred so far. Possible problems could be (see also Section 7.5.5, page 109):

- Lower than expected recruitment rate for studies of humans (researchers should explain the reasons for this, and what measures they have taken or plan to take to overcome this, including contact with centres with very few or no subjects).
- Administrative or logistical difficulties in obtaining approvals for studies at some or all participating centres.
- Protracted negotiations with commercial companies, for example, over the supply of free drugs or medical devices for a clinical trial, or free materials or equipment for laboratory studies.
- Unforeseen technical or methodological problems in a laboratory experiment, that may require it to be redesigned.

Even if a major problem occurs, it is still worthwhile highlighting any substantial achievements attained in the previous year.

If the study has an independent oversight committee (e.g. IDMC or TSC, see page 21), they should meet before the annual report is submitted to the funding body (in person or by teleconference). The oversight committee can examine the problems in detail, and often suggest potential solutions. Importantly, they can also provide a letter of support for continuing the study and give their approval for major changes to the study design, which can then be enclosed with the annual report.

In rare circumstances, the funding body will decide to terminate the study early in view of a highly unsatisfactory report. An obvious reason would be very poor recruitment, despite the study being open for several years. Even though money has already been allocated and used up, the funding committee may decide that it is not cost-effective to continue financing a study that clearly is unable to address its original objectives. If this does occur, the research team may still continue with the study, but they will have to find funds for this elsewhere.

8.2 Applying for a grant extension

A grant extension is treated in a similar way to a new grant application, and many funding bodies either have a specific form for this, or the researchers need to complete the standard application form for new project proposals (many of the features discussed in previous chapters apply). An extension may be sought if the original grant amount is not sufficient for the study to continue, either as planned or with a change to the design. Sometimes, an extension could have been avoided if the applicants provided more realistic costs in the original grant application. There are several reasons for extending a study, for example:

- The recruitment period needs to be extended because accrual is much slower than expected.
- The follow-up period needs to be extended in order to record enough events (e.g. deaths) for a reliable statistical analysis.
- The design needs to change (e.g. an increase in the target sample size).
- The study has taken much longer than expected to set up, due to unforeseen administrative or logistical issues, so the whole study duration has to be extended.
- For laboratory experiments, there could be serious problems with equipment, or the initial parts of the experiment may have produced unexpected results, meaning that subsequent stages are difficult to start or need to be redesigned.

If a grant extension is required, it is advisable for researchers to contact the administrative staff at the funding body to seek preliminary advice on how to proceed, before any application is submitted.

Researchers must provide a clear account of the problem(s), and explain how they might be resolved, or give reasons for extending the study in the application with a full justification. It is a mistake to believe that because a grant has already been awarded for a study, a request for an extension, which involves more money, will be automatically approved. This is not the case, particularly if there are many new applications being submitted, and bearing in mind that funding bodies have limited resources. The extension application will be competing with new study proposals, including those which might have a better chance of completing, have greater scientific interest or would have a higher impact on clinical practice or public health policy.

It might be difficult to apply for an extension if money for staff and other resources were requested at a time when there was clearly little work being undertaken on the study. For example, if a cohort study has had a full-time (1.0 FTE) co-ordinator and half-time (0.5 FTE) data manager for the past 3 years, but only recruited 50 subjects out of a target of 500, the funding committee or internal reviewers will understandably query what these staff have been working on, because there have been relatively little data to manage. It would have been better for the applicants to have requested lower staff costs in previous years when they noticed problems with accrual, and to have delayed access to the full funds until a time when the recruitment is progressing well. However, this can be difficult to do when a person is in post, and it has not been possible to fund them from other sources. Sometimes, it is best to reduce the amount requested during the extended part of the study, and only request the minimum of funds (i.e. low staff costs and running expenses, if possible).

When reviewing a grant extension application, the funding committee (perhaps with external reviewers) will consider:
- How much of the grant has been used already? If £200K has been spent, it might not be effective to spend a further £300K if the study is unlikely to complete.
- Have there been any achievements? Even if there are problems or reasons for extending the study, the researchers should always try to specify what has been achieved so far.
- If the extension is awarded, is there a high chance of the study completing and meeting its objectives?

- If the extension is not awarded, what are the implications? Could the research group still continue with the study in some form?
- If the study duration is to be extended by several years, could it become outdated, might participating centres lose interest or new technologies make the study obsolete? Would the study still be of interest in several years' time?
- Is there strong support and approval from the IDMC or TSC? Applicants should provide a letter of support from the oversight committee(s), when available.

Where appropriate, the above issues should be described and addressed in the extension application.

After the committee meeting, there may be further comments by the applicants to address, before a final decision is made. If the extension is awarded, certain conditions may need to be met, and an update report might be requested within a year. Continuing major problems will increase the chance of the study grant being terminated early at a later date.

Summary points

- Be aware of the process for updating the funding body during the project, ensuring that timelines for submitting annual reports are met.
- In an annual report, always try to provide what key achievements have been made, in addition to any major problems encountered.
- If there are problems, always specify ways of how they are likely to be resolved.
- If the initial grant needs to be increased in order to complete the project, contact the administrative staff at the funding body for advice before submitting an extension application.
- Provide a full justification for extending the grant.
- Do not assume that a grant extension will be automatically awarded.

Bibliography

FDA 2007. Guidance for industry: clinical trial endpoints for the approval of cancer drugs and biologics. http://www.fda.gov/downloads/Drugs/GuidanceCompliance RegulatoryInformation/Guidances/ucm071590.pdf.

FDA Good Manufacturing Practice. http://www.fda.gov/Food/GuidanceCompliance RegulatoryInformation/CurrentGoodManufacturingPracticesCGMPs/default.htm.

Glasziou P, Irwig L, Bain C, Colditz G. Systematic reviews in health care. A practical guide. Cambridge University Press, UK, 2001.

Govaert TME, Thijs MCN, Masurel N, Sprenger MJW, Dinant GJ, Knottnerus JA. The efficacy of influenza vaccination in elderly individuals. JAMA 1994; 272(21):1661–5.

Hackshaw AK. A concise guide to clinical trials. First edition. Wiley-Blackwell, UK, 2009.

Hackshaw AK, Harmer C, Mallick U, Haq M, Franklyn J. ^{131}I activity for remnant ablation in patients with differentiated thyroid cancer: a systematic review. J Clin Endocrin Metab 2007;92(1):28–38.

Katz R. Biomarkers and surrogate markers: an FDA perspective. NeuroRx: J Am Soc Exp Neurother 2004;1:189–95.

Khan KS, Kunz R, Kleijnen J, Antes G. Systematic reviews to support evidence-based medicine. Royal Society of Medicine Press Ltd, UK, 2003.

MacMahon S, Collins R. Reliable assessment of the effects of treatment on mortality and major morbidity, II: observational studies. Lancet 2001;357:455–62.

Mallick U, Harmer C, Hackshaw A. The HiLo trial: a multicentre randomised trial of high- versus low-dose radioiodine, with or without recombinant human thyroid stimulating hormone, for remnant ablation after surgery for differentiated thyroid cancer. Clin Oncol 2008;20(5):325–6.

Medicines and Healthcare products Regulatory Agency (MHRA); GMP and GLP. http://www.mhra.gov.uk/Howweregulate/Medicines/Inspectionandstandards/ GoodManufacturingPractice/index.htm.
http://www.mhra.gov.uk/Howweregulate/Medicines/Inspectionandstandards/ GoodLaboratoryPractice/index.htm.

Pope C, Mays N (eds). Qualitative research in health care. BMJ Books, Blackwell Publishing, UK, 2006.

Rothman KJ. Epidemiology: an introduction. Oxford University Press, USA, 2002.

Silman AJ, MacFarlane GJ. Epidemiological studies: a practical guide. Second edition. Cambridge University Press, UK, 2002.

Temple R. Are surrogate markers adequate to assess cardiovascular disease drugs? JAMA 1999;282(8):790–5.

Whitehead J, Matsushita T. Stopping clinical trials because of treatment ineffectiveness: a comparison of a futility design with a method of stochastic curtailment. Stat Med 2003;22(5):677–87.

Yang OO. Guide to effective grant writing: how to write an affective NIH grant application. Springer, USA, 2005.

Sample size (free software available on the Internet or with an accompanying book, or commercially available software):

Case–control and cohort studies:

http://www.cdc.gov/EpiInfo/.

http://www.sph.emory.edu/~cdckms/sample%20size%202%20grps%20case%20 control.html.

All studies:

Dupont WD, Plummer WD. PS power and sample size program available for free on the Internet. Control Clin Trials 1997;18:274. http://ps-power-and-sample-size-calculation.software.informer.com/.

Machin D, Campbell MJ, Tan SB, Tan SH. Sample size tables for clinical studies. Third edition. Wiley-Blackwell, UK, 2009 [comes with accompanying CD].

PASS (Power Analysis and Sample Size software). http://www.ncss.com/pass.html.

nQuery. http://www.statsol.ie/html/nquery/nquery_home.html.

Bibliography

Index